SWIRE'S HANDBOOK OF PRACTICAL NURSING

Swire's Handbook of
PRACTICAL NURSING

SIXTH EDITION REVISED
BY
Joan Burr
R.M.N., S.R.N.

*King's Fund Administrative Course, Formerly Deputy Matron
The Bethlem Royal and Maudsley Hospitals, and Deputy Principal
of the King's Fund Staff College for Ward Sisters*

BAILLIÈRE TINDALL & CASSELL
LONDON

First published as *Swire's Handbook for the Assistant Nurse*
1949
Second edition 1953
Third edition 1956
Fourth edition 1959

Reprinted as *Swire's Handbook for the Enrolled Nurse*
1961
Reprinted 1963
Fifth edition 1964
Reprinted 1966

Sixth edition published as *Swire's Handbook of Practical Nursing*
1968

SBN 7020-0268-2

Made and printed in Great Britain by
Cox & Wyman Ltd, London, Fakenham and Reading

Contents

Contents

PLATES

Preface

Miss Swire, who wrote the first edition of this well-known and widely used textbook, did so because at that time (1949) a new kind of nurse training was being devised in this country and no suitable book was available. It had become clear that there was a need and a place for nurses who had learnt their skill largely at the bedside and who did not require the extensive theoretical background which for the State Registered Nurse is essential. Since that time in other countries too the need for practical nurses has become apparent, and today they are hard at work in almost every country in the world—albeit under a variety of names.

In this country the practical nurse—the Enrolled Nurse—is to be found in almost every hospital and she is playing an indispensable part in the nursing care of the sick. Though she receives her training mainly at the bedside it is nevertheless necessary that she should have a textbook containing information on such subjects as, for example, anatomy and physiology. It was for this reason that Miss Swire wrote her book and Miss R. T. Farnol later undertook the task of revising and keeping up to date the information it contained as new editions were called for. 'This book,' as Miss Farnol wrote in her preface to the fifth edition, 'is the pupil nurse's own special book, which gives her the basic knowledge of the many subjects she has to learn in training.'

I was very pleased when I was asked to prepare a new sixth edition of this valuable textbook. Generally the major changes I

Preface

have made have been in approach. The book now opens with the section on Personal and Community Health as it is desirable that the nurse should be introduced to the principles governing health before her attention is directed towards disease. The chapter on the National Health Service has been considerably enlarged to include a description of the work done by the health visitor, mid-wife, home nurse, occupational health nurse and mental welfare officer, and of the part played by child guidance clinics, the school health service, meals on wheels, home helps and the ambulance service. It also gives in simple language an outline of human development from birth to old age. This is followed by The Patient in Hospital which has been re-arranged and carefully revised. The chapter on Nurse–Patient Relationship has been much enlarged. It now gives an introduction to human behaviour in illness and also touches on some of the emotional problems confronting the nurse in the course of her work. In response to the increasing importance attached to skilled geriatric nursing the chapter on Caring for the Elderly now deals in considerably more detail with both the physical and emotional aspects of this type of work. Anatomy and Physiology follows as the third section because it was thought that, although important, it did not now warrant the prominence accorded to it in previous editions.

I feel sure that this book will continue to prove a valuable text-book for enrolled nurses and for other practical nurses throughout the world as it contains the information they require and is clearly written in simple language. I hope also that it will continue to be of assistance to many Pupil Nurses and to overseas nurses, wherever they may train.

JOAN BURR

I

The Practical Nurse

Illness is as old as mankind. All through the ages sick people have needed nursing. When people hear the word 'nurse' they generally think of someone who knows what to do in an emergency, and does it with skill and compassion; someone who can soothe a feverish child, comfort a bereaved husband, or cheer the weariness of long term illness. Above all they think of someone whose hands bring relief and comfort to a sick person.

The practical nurse is the nurse at the patient's bedside. She is the person on whom the doctor relies to carry out his instructions with expert skill and understanding, whether the patient is in a hospital ward, a jungle village, a remote outpost, or a city slum. In some parts of the world she will be working side by side with her colleagues in the health team, but in others she may be separated from them by many miles, and the people she serves will look to her not only for nursing care but for education in the basic rules of personal and community health.

Her training shows her that unless people eat a properly balanced diet they will suffer from disease, whether it be kwashiorkor in the tropics, beriberi in the rice fields, or chronic infection in a bed-sitting room in Manchester. She knows that a pure water supply is vital to health, and that polluted water brings typhoid and dysentery in a London suburb as surely as it does in an African village. Her enemies may be mosquitoes and parasitic worms in the jungle, lice and bedbugs in a tenement, soft living in the stockbroker belt, or neurosis in a skyscraper, but all over the world she meets the same need for basic nursing care and health education.

For a long time nursing care was provided, in Britain, by the patient's relatives, by members of religious communities, or by women who were hired for the job but were untrained and generally quite unsuitable for the work. It was the vision and determination of Florence Nightingale, at the end of the nineteenth century, which finally won recognition for British nurses and established their right to a proper training.

Today two types of training are available in the British Isles. One prepares nurses to qualify for registration, and the other to qualify for enrolment. The Register and the Roll are both maintained by the General Nursing Council, which also regulates the training of nurses and their examinations in this country. In other countries similar training is given, in addition to that for registration, as for example in Australia, where the nurses we call 'Enrolled Nurses' are called 'Nursing Aides'.

The registered nurse carries the responsibility of administering the ward, organizing the work of other nurses, teaching and leading the ward team, but the enrolled nurse has the satisfaction of being free from administration and able to give her whole attention to the practical nursing care of the patient. She learns her work principally at the bedside, with some theoretical training in the classroom. Her training can take place in many different kinds of hospital. She may have experience in nursing acutely ill patients, sick children, psychiatric patients, the elderly sick, and may work in special departments such as the operating theatre or the out-patient department.

The demand for enrolled nurses is greatly in excess of the supply, and will continue to grow. At the same time many opportunities are now open to enrolled nurses who want to take further training, or to work in the community. Modern nursing needs both registered and enrolled nurses. Working together they can offer the comprehensive nursing care which the patient needs, and the good enrolled nurse is recognized as one of the most valuable members of the ward team.

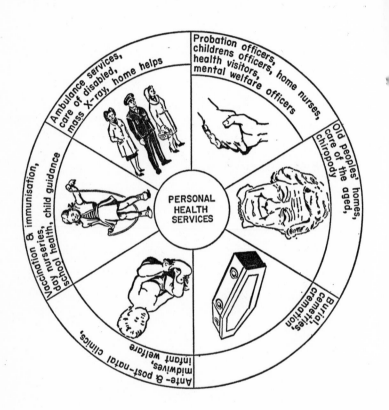

Probation officers, childrens officers, home nurses, health visitors, mental welfare officers

Old peoples' homes, care of the aged, chiropody

Burial, cemetries, cremation

Ante- & post-natal clinics, midwives, infant welfare

Vaccination & immunisation, day nurseries, child guidance school health,

Ambulance services, care of disabled, mass X-ray, home helps

PERSONAL HEALTH SERVICES

Personal and Community Health

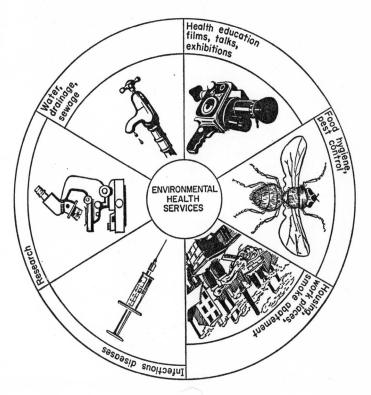

Health education films, talks, exhibitions

Water, drainage, sewage

Food hygiene, pest control

ENVIRONMENTAL HEALTH SERVICES

Research

Housing, work places, smoke abatement

Infectious diseases

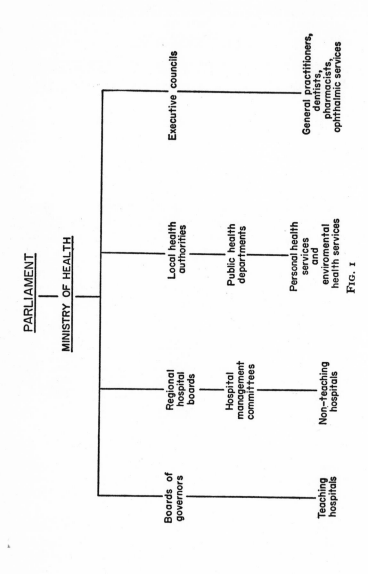

PARLIAMENT

MINISTRY OF HEALTH

Boards of governors — Regional hospital boards — Local health authorities — Executive councils

Hospital management committees

Public health departments

Teaching hospitals — Non-teaching hospitals — Personal health services and enviromental health services — General practitioners, dentists, pharmacists, ophthalmic services

FIG. I

2

The National Health Service

We have a comprehensive Health Service in Britain which cares for the health of everyone in the community and provides services to deal with every kind of health problem from before birth, through childhood and adolescence, to maturity and old age. In some, but not all, other countries there are various other forms of health service, but this chapter deals only with the health service that exists in this country today.

The head of the National Health Service in Great Britain is the Minister of Health, who is accountable to Parliament. The Minister has a Chief Nursing Officer and a Chief Medical Officer to advise him, and, of course, a very large staff.

The Minister gives the job of running the hospitals to the Regional Hospital Boards, of which there are fifteen all over the country.

The Regional Hospital Boards take the hospitals in their areas and divide them up into groups. Then they put a Hospital Management Committee in charge of each group. It is the Hospital Management Committee which is responsible for the day to day running of the hospital.

An exception is made in the case of teaching hospitals, which are hospitals used for the training of doctors. Teaching hospitals are run by Boards of Governors, not by Regional Hospital Boards.

The general practitioners, dentists, pharmacists and ophthalmic services are governed by Executive Councils in each area, and public health is the responsibility of the Local Health Authorities.

Public health departments can be divided into those concerned with promoting personal health and those concerned with providing a healthy environment for people to live in. The head of the public health department is the Medical Officer of Health for each area.

Some of the ways in which people can be helped by the National Health Service are described below.

Maternity Care

John and Mary Smith had been married eighteen months, and when Mary knew that she was going to have a baby they were both delighted.

Mary's general practitioner arranged for her to attend the ante-natal clinic every month, and here she met the midwife and the health visitor who would look after her and the baby. On her first visit the clinic doctor gave her a thorough examination and told her that everything was satisfactory.

Mary enjoyed the meetings at the clinic. There were several girls like herself who were expecting their first babies, and some older women who already had one or two children. Although she was pleased to be having the baby Mary couldn't help feeling a little scared at first. She remembered some of the talk she had overheard as a child between her mother and Aunt Gladys, and she hoped it wouldn't be quite as bad as that. But as the months went by she found her fears dissolving as she joined in the friendly discussions with the nurses and the other women at the clinic.

She learnt how important it was to eat plenty of protein, fresh vegetables, fruit and milk, to give the growing baby a really healthy start, and the nurses gave her concentrated orange juice and vitamin tablets to supplement the vitamins in her own food. She also attended relaxation classes in preparation for the birth.

As everything was straightforward the doctor decided that

6

Mary could have her baby at home. All went well, and the mid-wife from the clinic, who was an old friend by now, said that baby Alan was a first class specimen. She continued to look after Mary and the baby for the next two weeks until Mary felt quite happy about feeding, bathing and caring for little Alan, and was strong enough to carry on by herself.

John was overjoyed to see Mary so well. He soon began to take an interest in Alan's routine and became quite expert at bathing and changing nappies.

The Health Visitor

Health visitors are responsible, among many things, for the care of children until they are five years old, and at the end of two weeks the health visitor from the clinic came to see Alan and had a friendly chat with Mary and John. She said she would be dropping in from time to time to see how they were getting on and Mary was glad to know that here was someone she could turn to if she felt at all worried.

On the health visitor's advice Mary took Alan regularly to the infant welfare clinic where his progress was assessed, and it was here that he was immunized against diphtheria, tetanus and whooping cough, and vaccinated against smallpox. Mary was a bit doubtful as to whether this was necessary because no one ever had diphtheria these days, but the health visitor explained that it was only through widespread immunization that these dangerous diseases had been brought under control. If immunization was stopped diphtheria would be back in no time.

Little Alan grew quickly. He really was a beautiful baby and there was no doubt he was the centre of Mary's world. 'You and that baby!' laughed her sister, 'Anyone would think you were the only woman ever to have one!'

Next to food a young baby needs love more than anything else. Its mother is its whole world and a warm, happy relationship with her during the early years is the best preparation any child can have for a normal, satisfying adult life later on. No wonder Alan was thriving. But there was a wistful look on John's face sometimes as he watched them together. He couldn't help thinking of the evenings when he and Mary used to go out, before Alan came. Surely it wouldn't do any harm to have a babysitter just once in a while? But Mary wouldn't hear of it.

Alan was three years old when Mary found she was pregnant again. She was a bit daunted at the thought of another baby but the months passed quickly and soon Alan was joined by his little sister, Christine.

There were many times now when, instead of being with him all the time, Mary had to leave Alan to his own devices while she attended to Christine. It was hard work looking after the two of them, and the house, and the shopping, and the cooking, and everything. John didn't seem to realize how much there was to do and how tired she felt in the evenings.

To make matters worse Alan started bedwetting. He was difficult to handle too, and Mary was afraid his screaming would upset the neighbours.

For some time John and Mary had been having arguments. It started over the children, but lately it seemed to Mary they had been quarrelling about everything. She felt so depressed that the next time the health visitor came she poured it all out to her.

The health visitor seemed to understand exactly how Mary felt, and she asked if she could come back when John was home from work and have a talk with them both.

When they were all together she explained that Alan was perfectly normal but he was jealous because he thought his mother had stopped loving him now that she had Christine. Because he couldn't put his feelings into words he was trying to get her attention back by bedwetting and temper tantrums.

John and Mary found it was a relief to talk to the health visitor, and they were thankful to know that Alan's behaviour was quite natural. The health visitor told them that he would soon get over it if Mary could show him that she did still love him. Perhaps one of the best ways would be to let him 'help' her in looking after Christine.

John soon realized that Alan wasn't the only one who was jealous. He saw now that he, himself, had actually been jealous of his own baby son at times, because he seemed to claim all Mary's love and affection.

The health visitor said this too was quite natural, and often happened to young couples when children came along. The thing to do was to talk to one another about it openly, and not keep it all bottled up inside.

Alan soon stopped bedwetting when Mary divided her attention more fairly between the children. She also agreed to leave them with a neighbour once a week, so that she and John could go out together. 'It's fine!'—'Just like old times,' said John. He and Mary could laugh about it now, but it had been pretty serious at the time.

Landmarks in Human Development

There are certain landmarks in the growth of a human being, and one of the first is the arrival of a brother or sister. For the first time the child has to share his mother, who means everything to him, with a stranger. It can even seem that she thinks more of this stranger than she does of him. If the trouble is not recognized at this stage he may grow up with a secret fear that he is somehow not quite as good as other people. Many an eldest child unconsciously spends his life striving to prove that he is better than the next man because he has this doubt about his own value.

Other landmarks are going to school, puberty and adolescence, going to work, marriage, middle age, retirement, and old age. At each stage the human being can take another step forward in his development, or, if the stress is too much for him, he may become ill, either physically, or mentally, or both.

Child guidance clinics

For children who are emotionally upset and do not respond as well as Alan did there are special child guidance clinics. These are run by a child psychiatrist, a psychiatric social worker and a psychologist.

The psychologist uses tests to discover the child's level of intelligence and the extent of his emotional disturbance. The psychiatric social worker investigates his background and talks to his parents. They both report to the child psychiatrist, who is a doctor specializing in the mental illnesses of childhood, and he advises the parents on the treatment needed.

School Health

Going to school was rather frightening at first, but Alan soon began to enjoy it. Mixing with the other children made him less dependent on his mother and he grew into a sturdy, adventurous youngster.

The health of children at school is the concern of the school nurse and the school doctor, who is often the Medical Officer of Health for the area. Together they carry out regular examinations of the children. Eyes, ears, teeth, mental and physical development, all receive attention and help is given where necessary.

All children have free milk because it is such a complete food, and those who remain at school at midday are given well planned meals, containing plenty of the protein and vitamins which growing children need so much.

Special schools

There are special schools for children who are physically handicapped, e.g. for blind, deaf, or spastic children. Mentally ill children are generally treated at the child guidance clinic but some may be sent to special schools. Some children have minds which cannot develop beyond a certain point. They are called mentally sub-normal and there are special schools for them also.

Because of the care given through the school health service it is often at school that the first signs of mental or physical ill health are noticed. The health visitor and school nurse play an important part in the service because they provide a link between the school and the parents.

Adolescence

Mary found that the health visitor gave talks at the school on various aspects of health, including sex education. Some of these were for the children and others for their parents. Mary and John went as often as they could. They found them a great help when it came to answering questions from Alan and Christine, and preparing them for the changes that puberty would bring. Later on, when the children were in their teens, Mary found that looking back on these talks helped her to understand them a little better when they were moody and difficult.

Puberty and adolescence is a time of rapid change and growth both physically and emotionally. A few young people go through this period with no apparent stress, but for the majority it is a time of great heart searching. Rebellion against parents is natural. Nature wants the fledgling to leave the nest and try its wings. Also natural is an intense interest in the opposite sex. Waywardness, idealism, depression, hero worship, sudden enthusiasms and boredom are all common. The adolescent is an adult one moment and a child the next. What he needs more than anything else is simple, warm, unwavering affection.

A very small proportion of adolescents become delinquents, but the majority grow into mature men and women able to enjoy a normal life.

Occupational Health

Leaving school and going to work was a big change for Alan. At school he had done well and had been given quite a lot of responsibility during his last year. He was also good at games and something of a hero to the younger children, but when he went as an apprentice to the large engineering works on the other side of the town all this changed overnight.

Here he was very small fry. The men took no notice of him except to tell him briefly what to do. The women eyed him up and down and teased him. The other apprentices were not too bad, but even they made it plain that he was the junior and the dogsbody.

He soon began to find his feet, however, and discovered, to his surprise, that the men were keen to help him, the women were good fun, and some of the other apprentices were ready to make friends. But a few young people, not as stable as Alan, find difficulty in adjusting to the demands of this new situation and it is often the occupational health nurse who is the first to notice this.

The health of workers in large industrial organizations is the concern of the works doctor and the occupational health nurse.

Factories and workshops are required by law to conform to a set standard for lighting, heating, ventilation, work space, lavatory accommodation, wash-rooms and canteens, and stringent safety precautions are enforced. Major disasters are rare and the bulk of the physical treatments carried out in the works surgery are for minor cuts and bruises, coughs and colds, stomach upsets, backaches and so on.

The occupational health nurse also helps workers with emotional problems, worries over home conditions, family misunderstandings, arguments with workmates, disagreements with the management, fears of redundancy, hopes of promotion—they all find their way to the surgery on some pretext or another, and she can play a large part in preventing absenteeism and in promoting good relationships in the organization.

Middle Age

For John and Mary the years passed quickly and in no time at all Alan was married, with a son of his own, while Christine was doing well as an enrolled nurse and sharing a flat with a friend from the same hospital.

Now that the children were off their hands John and Mary had much more time to themselves. For some people this stage in their lives can be difficult. For a long time they look forward to being free, having a little peace and quiet, being able to go out and enjoy themselves without worrying about the children, having the house to themselves, and so on. But somehow it doesn't work out like this. Everything seems flat. There's no point in doing anything. Although they don't realize it the truth is they feel useless now that the children have gone.

Often this time coincides with the start of the menopause (the change of life) for the wife. Now that she is losing her ability to bear children she feels that she is somehow losing her femininity as well, and may no longer be attractive to her husband. A few women become so depressed at this time that they need a short stay in hospital for psychiatric treatment, but fortunately most couples pass through this stage without great difficulty.

John and Mary had always thought they would like to have a bungalow by the sea, near to John's mother and father, and they wisely decided that it was better to move now, while they had plenty of time to make new friends and put down fresh roots before they retired, rather than to wait until they were older when they might feel less inclined to face the upheaval.

John's parents were in their late seventies. His mother was handicapped by arthritis and his father's heart was none too good, but all the same they managed to enjoy life. Mr Smith had some tablets for his heart, which he took every day, and once a week the ambulance came and took Mrs Smith to hospital for her treatment.

Between them they could manage to get washed and dressed in the morning, and light meals were not too difficult to cope with. But general cooking and housework had become too much for them, and of course shopping was a problem because Mr Smith couldn't walk far enough to reach the shops and Mrs Smith was too handicapped by her arthritis to carry a shopping bag.

They had explained the difficulty to their doctor and he had arranged for a home help to come twice a week to do the shopping and housework. The meals on wheels service called on three days and left them a good hot meal, and every Friday the district nurse came and helped them each to have a bath.

John and Mary frequently went over to see them and on one occasion the health visitor was there. Mrs Smith introduced John and Mary, and as they all sat talking together the health visitor explained that it was part of her job to keep an eye on old people as well as on children. In fact, she said, a health visitor looks after the whole family, and her aim is to promote good health in all its aspects, both physically and mentally.

The district nurse

The district nurse looks after people who have recently been discharged from hospital and perhaps have wounds to be dressed, or need injections. She also cares for handicapped people and old people like Mr and Mrs Smith who need help in taking a bath, cutting their nails, or in any other details of their personal care.

Home helps and meals on wheels

John and Mary were also interested in the home help and in the meals on wheels service, and the health visitor told them that home helps were employed by the local health authority to give domestic help in households where she, or the district nurse, or the general practitioner thought it was necessary. They did shopping, cleaning, cooking, washing, and looked after the children. They were often called in to give help to old people like Mr and Mrs Smith, and also for short periods when a mother might be ill in hospital or having another baby, and father and the children could not manage on their own.

The meals on wheels service, run by the Women's Royal Voluntary Service, also gave invaluable help by providing hot nourishing meals for people unable to cook for themselves, and again it would be the nurses or the general practitioner who arranged this.

The mental welfare officer

As they sat talking Mr and Mrs Smith told them that two doors away the daughter of the house had been in a psychiatric hospital for two months, earlier in the year. She was at home now and 'the man from the welfare' came to see her each week.

This, said the health visitor, was another of her colleagues, the mental welfare officer, whose special job was to help people who were mentally ill. 'In fact,' she said, 'all of us in the National Health Service, whether we are based in hospital or out in the community, try to work together as a team, so that we can give a really all round service.'

Retirement and Old Age

John and Mary made many friends in their new district and they also became interested in some of the voluntary work which was being done locally. John joined the staff of a youth club and found he had quite a gift for handling young boys and girls. Mary had always felt concerned about handicapped people who could not get out and must, she felt, be desperately lonely at times. She mentioned this at church one day and in no time she had a small group of people to visit. One was a young man paralysed as the result of a road accident, another was a woman of 43 who had multiple sclerosis, and then there was an old man with an artificial leg and an elderly woman who was partially blind. Mary soon got to know them and became deeply interested in what she called her 'new family'.

Life was full and enjoyable, and John really began to look forward to the time when he could retire. Not that he didn't enjoy his work, but there were so many other things he wanted to do that his leisure never seemed long enough.

Many people, finding the responsibility of their work weighs heavy, or tired with the monotony of routine, sigh for the day when they can give it all up and do nothing. But doing literally nothing palls quickly, and their pleasure in getting up late each morning and sitting in the garden all day soon turns to an uneasy feeling that life is passing them by, they are the have-beens who no longer make any contribution to the life of the world. It is only a short step from this feeling to a state of apathy and depression in which nothing seems worth doing anyway.

Retirement and old age can be a time of real stress unless it is planned in advance and filled with worthwhile, satisfying activity, but for people like John and Mary it is truly a time of fulfilment when, as mature men and women, they can use their talents to the full and make happy relationships with those of a younger generation as well as with their contemporaries.

Alan and Christine looked forward to visiting their parents. So did Alan's wife Sara and their young son Jimmy. 'There'll always be a place for you in our house if you want it,' said Sara, smiling at her mother-in-law. 'It would be fun having you with us!'

From this short account of an imaginary family we can see that the National Health Service provides many services and employs specially trained people to run them, so as to help us in time of need at every stage of our lives from earliest childhood to old age. It is extremely important that every nurse should be aware of these services since each patient and each patient's family is entitled to receive the full benefits of them.

3

The Health of the Community

For proper development both of mind and body, and for the maintenance of health, certain laws must be obeyed, otherwise the powers of resistance to disease weaken and health rapidly deteriorates.

People live longer now, and children are bonnier and healthier than they have ever been. Old people are better cared for, and sick ones return to their work quicker than ever before.

Moreover, since it is impossible for anyone to live an isolated existence and keep the consequences of his actions entirely to himself, the law must protect the whole community by enforcing penalties upon those who make of themselves either a public nuisance or a danger.

That is one reason why plans for new buildings must be submitted to the Local Authority, for approval of the *construction*, *drainage system* and *water supply*, why public health inspectors are appointed, and why health visitors are sent to advise people in their homes.

More and more it is being realized that disease and disability should not occur and that preventive measures, e.g. health education and clinics, are much better and more economical than curative treatments. Good health and the wellbeing of the individual and the community, demand that people should:

1. Breathe pure air. The law lays down regulations about the ventilation of the places where people live and work.
2. Eat wholesome food in correct quantities and at regular intervals.
3. Drink pure water and safe milk.
4. Wear clothing adapted to climate and occupation.
5. Live in properly constructed and suitably placed houses.
6. Have as much sunshine and fresh air as possible.
7. Cultivate good habits and obtain enough rest and sleep in a well-ventilated bedroom.
8. Secure enjoyable recreation which rests and broadens the mind, and suitable exercise which benefits and develops all the systems of the body.

Of course, there is still a great deal to be done. There are still slums, and there are still underfed people, but every year sees some advance in the fight against poverty and ignorance.

Air

Fresh air is necessary for the healthy functioning of the body.

Air contains:

79% nitrogen
20% oxygen
0·04% carbon dioxide
Water vapour and various impurities

Air may be contaminated by:

1. Smoke from coal fires and factory chimneys.
2. Petrol/oil fumes from motor vehicles.
3. Tobacco smoke.
4. Chemicals from factory wastes.
5. Dust, soot and grit.
6. Droplet infection, i.e. germs spread by sneezing and coughing.
7. Carbon dioxide from the breath of men and animals.

Air is purified by :

1. Sunlight, which kills germs.
2. Rain, which washes away some impurities.
3. Frost, which prevents the growth of germs.
4. The green colouring matter in plants called chlorophyll. This enables the plant to take the carbon dioxide in the air, which is a poison to us, to use the carbon out of it as a food, and to release the oxygen, which we need.

Fog and smog. Sometimes a layer of cold air, heavy with water vapour, lies over the earth quite low down. If it cannot move because there is no wind, it gathers more and more impurities from smoke, petrol fumes, soot, sulphur, etc., until we can see it and feel it. It may become so dense that it envelops everything, shutting out the sunlight and pure air above. This is what we call smog and it occurs over big cities. Fog is a similar condition occurring over country districts also but is not quite so laden with impurities.

All this is bad enough for healthy people, but for those already suffering from chest complaints it can be fatal.

The Clean Air Act came into force in the winter of 1956, making it an offence in towns to use fuel which gives off dark smoke. Special smokeless fuel has to be used. There are means of tracing where smoke is coming from, and how much.

Ventilation

It is the duty of every nurse to see that her patient's room is well ventilated and that there are no draughts.

The harmful effects of a badly ventilated room are due to the fact that the moisture and heat given off from the occupants' bodies makes the air overheated and damp, and so prevents the lungs and skin from functioning properly. Consequently the waste products of the body are retained and symptoms of headache, nausea, loss of appetite and depression, arise. There is also a tendency to faintness and an increased liability to contract infection.

Ventilation may depend on:

1. The action of winds.
2. The movement of gases in the atmosphere, which is utilized in the ventilation of buildings by means of *inlets* and *outlets*, the commonest form of inlet being the window and the commonest forms of outlet being the chimney, or fans which suck air out (in modern blocks of flats for example).

Draughts may often be avoided by raising the lower sash of a window and placing a board across it so that the air enters in an upward direction.

Special perforated bricks in walls, or panes of glass in windows are sometimes included during building, so that air can come in and go out even when it is too cold or windy to have the windows open. If you look around your own hospital you may find some of these devices.

Artificial ventilation is a feature of the great blocks of new offices, factories and public buildings that are going up today. In hospitals you will find it in the operating theatres and in certain wards. Air is drawn in by strong fans, and then 'conditioned', i.e. it is filtered of impurities, heated or cooled, and made more or less moist or dry according to the requirements of the occupants. It then circulates through the building and is sucked out by another mechanism. Some people find this kind of 'pre-packed' air rather tiring and depressing, and prefer the draughts and extra work of the old-fashioned windows!

On the other hand, ventilation may be secured by a system of fans and ducts designed to propel fresh air into a building and forcibly draw out the impure air.

Light and Lighting

Sunlight and fresh air are very beneficial to health and the ultra-violet rays of the sun are effective in killing germs. Windows should be kept clean and should be arranged so that the lighting in a room will enable a person with normal eyesight to read ordinary print in any corner of the room.

In lighting, *glare* should be avoided, and when writing or working the light should fall from the left side.

Forms of artificial lighting

Paraffin oil lamps, although cheap, and the only method available in some country districts, can be dangerous and give off impurities in the form of carbon dioxide and water.

Coal gas to some extent uses up the oxygen in the air of a room.

Electric light is generally more expensive than gas lighting but gives off no impurities and uses up no oxygen.

Lamps should be shaded to avoid glare. It should be remembered that a lamp filament is very brittle, so lampshades, etc., must be dusted very carefully.

Heating

We keep warm by:

> Wearing clothes
> Living in houses
> Using artificial heating

The open fire is bright and cheerful and is a good ventilator, but except in the more modern grates it is extravagant as much of the heat is wasted. *Stoves* should have a flue. They are economical but their ventilating effect is less than that of an open fire. For both of these only smokeless fuels may be used in the smokeless zones.

Radiators and pipes should be well dusted and protected by wire guards.

Gas fires are clean, convenient and easily regulated, but they have a drying effect on the air.

Electric radiators and electric fires are excellent but expensive to run.

Central heating, by water or steam, or a combination of oil and electricity, is the most economical and effective method of heating larger buildings. Sometimes the pipes are hidden in the walls, and sometimes under the floor boards to give an evenly distributed warmth.

The comfortable temperature for a ward is about 18·5° C (65° F). A surgical ward may be a bit warmer, while the operating theatre will be kept at about 22° C (70° F). The under-floor system is used in some hospital wards and theatres.

Water

Water is a chemical compound of hydrogen and oxygen. About 40 gallons per head a day are needed for personal and public use. Water comes from the rainfall by:

1. Evaporation from wet surfaces, lakes, ponds, etc., and then falling again as rain.
2. Penetration into the soil and forming wells and springs.
3. Streams and rivers.

Pure water comes from upland lakes and reservoirs, and from deep and artesian wells. Impure water is that drawn from rivers and shallow wells.

A water supply may be contaminated by leaking pipes, by soft water acting on lead pipes and by pollution with sewage from leaking cesspools.

Diseases which may be caused by impure water are:

> Dysentery
> Parasitic diseases, e.g. worms
> Diarrhoea
> Cholera
> Typhoid and paratyphoid fever

Good *drinking water* should be pure, clear and sparkling, free from odour, taste and deposits, and it must not be so 'soft' as to dissolve lead, otherwise the water carried in lead pipes may lead to lead-poisoning.

Our water supply is one of the best in the world, and is purified for every town and village at special centres, where the water goes through prolonged filtration aided by natural and chemical means until it can pass the strictest tests for purity. It is then stored in great tanks and reservoirs until it is drawn off in the main pipes to serve houses, hospitals, and buildings everywhere.

All these processes cost a great deal of our money in the form of rates, especially to big concerns like hospitals, so nurses should play their part in preventing waste by turning off all taps carefully, being moderate with their bath water (do *not* let it overflow!), and reporting faulty washers and leaking taps.

The Disposal of Refuse

House refuse should either be burned or wrapped in a newspaper so as not to attract flies, then placed in a galvanized iron or plastic dustbin with a lid.

The Local Sanitary Authority is responsible for the emptying of dustbins once a week.

Rubbish may be tipped into the sea, at points where the tide will not wash it back. In some places, it is dumped on special areas of waste ground.

Offensive matter such as carcasses may be burned in a furnace. Clinker, the dust from the furnace, is sometimes used for trade purposes and the heat from the burning refuse for generating steam.

Metal is separated from the rubbish and sold as scrap.

Broken crockery may be used for filling up uneven ground.

Bones may be used for manure and rags may be sterilized and used for making paper.

Hospital refuse contains innumerable germs, so it should always be burned. Soiled dressings and tow, etc., are placed directly into a disposal bag at the bedside. The bag is sealed at once and placed in the soiled dressings bin. The bins are collected by a porter, their contents burnt, and the bins themselves are sterilized and returned to the ward. If disposal bags are not available it is a good idea to line the bin with a strong paper bag or with newspaper to reduce the risk of infection when the bin is being emptied. Make certain that no glass ever gets into the soiled dressings bin. It may injure the person emptying it.

Human excreta is removed by the water carriage system, but a chemical closet such as the 'Elsan' may be necessary in some remote districts, and of course, in caravans. The manufacturers of these closets supply a chemical preparation to dissolve the excreta so that it can be disposed of easily.

In the water carriage system, the contents of lavatory pans are flushed into a drain and then into a sewer. Where there are no sewers a cesspool is used instead. This is made of brick lined with cement and is placed at a safe distance from houses and streams. It is emptied periodically by the authorities.

The lavatory pan should be of smooth, glazed material and the back should be straight to prevent fouling.

The bottom end of the pan has a trap, that is a bend in the pipe, and this contains 2 inches of water known as the 'water seal' which prevents foul air from the drain from entering the building. Traps are provided with a movable inspection fitment so that any obstruction can easily be removed.

Lavatory pans discharge their contents into a *soil pipe,* the top end of which is always carried above the eaves with its open end protected by a wire cage to prevent birds from building their nests in it. Its lower end passes straight through the ground into the *house drain.* Waste water from baths and sinks is removed by the *waste pipe* which is separated from the house drain by a trap known as a gully.

A *manhole* is placed where the house drain empties into the street sewer. This contains a raking arm for cleaning purposes and a ventilator constructed in such a way that the impure air from the drain is prevented from escaping. Sewage disposal is a long and complicated process which ends in the complete purification of everything brought to the works.

At the sewage works, sewage passes through a *screen* made of iron bars in order to remove articles such as old mops and scrubbing brushes, etc., which may have been thrown down the drains. After the grit has been removed, the sewage passes into a tank where it is separated into:

1. A fluid part, or *effluent.*
2. A more solid part, the *sludge.*

Sludge may be dumped in the sea, if convenient, tipped on the land for use as manure (this is done free of charge) or burned in a destructor.

The *effluent* is treated so as to make it harmless, when it may be distributed over the soil or discharged into rivers. This fluid is tested at frequent intervals for the presence of bacteria. In this way germs such as those of typhoid fever can be detected and the whole effluent treated so that there will be no risk of any organisms passing on to endanger the water supply.

The site of a house or hospital should be as dry and warm as possible. For this reason, gravel and sand are the most suitable sites because these soils are porous.

The ground must be covered with a thick layer of concrete and between this and the floor there must be a space of at least 3 inches.

Walls should be 9 inches thick, and below the ground level there should be a cavity 2 to 3 inches wide, while a few inches above ground level there should be a *damp proof* course of impervious material such as asphalt or slate to prevent damp from rising up the walls. Rules are laid down by law regarding space, lighting, ventilation, drainage, water supply and general safety.

4

Household Pests and Parasites

People must be protected from *parasites*, i.e. animal and vegetable organisms which are dependent on the human body for their existence, and from *flies*, which spread disease owing to their habits of feeding on manure and garbage and then settling on food. All these creatures are enemies to health.

House Flies

The fly cannot eat solid food; it first dissolves it with its saliva, which it regurgitates on to it, and then sucks it up. It often vomits this again on to the food or elsewhere and defaecates while it is eating, and so contaminates food with germs. A fly's body is covered with hairs so that it is continually collecting dust. By means of adhesive pads on its feet, it can walk upside down.

Prevention of the spread of the fly nuisance
1. See that all dustbins, food buckets and rubbish pails are kept well covered and are regularly cleaned out and disinfected.
2. See that rubbish is removed frequently, because it takes only eight days for a fly to develop from an egg.
3. Keep all food covered and when laying tables place crockery upside down until it is used.

4. Cover larder windows with fine wire or gauze netting, so fresh air can get in but flies cannot.
5. Keep manure and compost heaps away from the house.

Lice, Fleas and Other Insects

The head louse is a little light-greyish insect with six legs. It lays its eggs, known as *nits*, in hard cases and deposits them on the hairs of the victim's head near the roots. The eggs hatch in about 10 days and the lice immediately begin to cause irritation by sucking blood.

Head lice are destroyed by the application of a preparation known as Suleo Hair Emulsion, which contains the insecticide DDT, used as directed on the bottle.

There are several other proprietary preparations on the market. These liquids are applied to the hair and scalp with a pipette, left on for a few hours, and then the hair is washed.

Carbolic acid and sassafras oil are unpleasant old fashioned remedies and should be used only when modern preparations are unobtainable.

The body louse is similar in appearance to the head louse. It is found on unclean and usually elderly people. Its colour changes according to the colour of the hair on the body of its victim. The nits are attached to the fibres of clothing by sticky substances.

Clothing must be disinfected by steam under pressure and ironed along the seams. The patient must have a hot bath, and *white precipitate* ointment or *sulphur* ointment is applied to the affected parts after thorough shaving.

Many diseases are caused by lice, among them *typhus* fever, fortunately now almost unknown in this country. Nurses, who protect themselves from lice by wearing protective clothing and who keep well, seldom contract the infection.

The flea has a horny brown skin and very large strong back legs for jumping. Fleas take about 19 days to develop and, if well fed, they may live for more than a year. They lay their eggs in beds and in cracks and crevices of a dirty room. Flea-infested rooms and articles must be fumigated by the Sanitary Authorities and all dust must be burned. To prevent fleas, it is absolutely essential to avoid all accumulations of rubbish, and to be scrupulously clean both in person and dwelling. Keating's insect powder is very useful and effective. This now contains DDT.

In Eastern countries there is also a variety of flea which may suck the blood of a rat infected with plague and so be the means of transmitting plague to human beings.

Rats may cause, in addition to plague, food poisoning, worms and jaundice, and they may be a source of danger to children and animals whom they are liable to attack.

If a rat is seen, the local Public Health Authorities should be told. They will send an expert to deal with these pests.

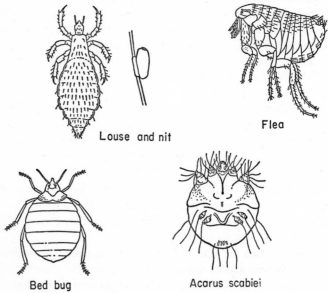

Louse and nit

Flea

Bed bug

Acarus scabiei

FIG. 2. COMMON PARASITES

The bed bug is a flat, oval, brownish-red insect. It lays its eggs in clusters in the cracks of old walls, floors and furniture, and these mature in about a week. Ordinary methods of fumigation are useless, therefore a special gas must be used, but only by *authorized* persons in *empty* premises, as this gas is *deadly* poison.

The itchmite, or *Acarus scabiei*. This parasite is a round, white, shiny, eyeless mite. It is very tiny but is just visible to the naked eye. It burrows deep into the thin parts of the skin, e.g. the crevices of the fingers, toes and elbows, and lays its eggs, then seals them up by means of a sticky fluid which it deposits all over the skin.

Treatment consists in gently scrubbing open the burrows when the patient has had a hot bath, killing the parasite by applying a preparation of benzyl benzoate, especially between the fingers and toes and all crevices. The emulsion is allowed to dry on before dressing, i.e. about 20 minutes. The patient must be given clean clothing after this application, and all clothing and bed linen used by him must be fumigated before it is washed. The mattress must be sent to be fumigated and the bedstead washed well with hot soapy water and disinfected.

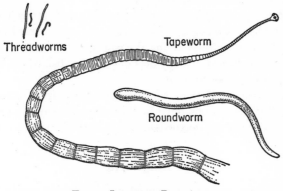

FIG. 3. INTERNAL PARASITES

Worms

Threadworms appear in the stools like little white threads with pointed heads and tails. They may be contracted by drinking infected water or by eating imperfectly prepared vegetables. It is therefore necessary, in the case of anyone suffering from threadworms, to see that the drinking water is boiled and that vegetables are well washed before they are cooked. Children are most commonly infested, and they are liable to reinfest themselves, and others around them, because the eggs of the worm are laid in the anus. They soon dry, and are freely dispersed in the clothing and on floors and carpets. The child will tend to scratch, and take the eggs to his mouth on his fingers. While treatment is going on it is essential that this be prevented by applying a soothing ointment to the anus, and lightly splinting the arms at night.

The roundworm is similar to the earthworm but paler in colour. It is from 6 to 16 inches long. Like the threadworm it may be due to infected water and vegetables. It may wander about the body causing disease and obstruction and may be vomited from the stomach or passed in the stools.

The symptoms of roundworm infestation are mostly abdominal pain and, in some cases, convulsions.

Tapeworms, which may be many feet long, consist of a head and a body which is made up of segments and which may break off from the head without killing the worm. They enter the body when infected meat (usually beef or pork), or fish which has not been properly cooked is eaten.

Treatment for all these worms is by special drugs ordered by the doctor. Directions must be carefully followed and all stools examined until the doctor is satisfied that the patient is cured.

Ringworm

Ringworm, or tinea, is caused by a vegetable mould (not a worm) which may attack either the scalp or the skin of the body. It forms spores, which if allowed to blow about, spread the infection wherever they settle. Cats are sometimes a means of spreading it. If there is reason to suspect a pet as the cause, it should be taken to a vet. Animals can be cured too.

Special methods are employed for detecting ringworm and the treatment may be by an antibiotic drug which is given by mouth, and seems to kill these fungi from inside the body, while fungicidal ointments are applied to the affected areas.

The linen must be changed daily and if hats are worn they should have a washable cotton lining.

Everything used by the patient must be thoroughly disinfected.

5

Milk and Food

Milk is one of the most important articles of food, especially for children. It contains all the factors necessary for life in proper proportion: proteins, carbohydrates, fats, mineral salts and vitamins and water.

Because it is the perfect food, germs find it so too, so unfortunately it is very easily contaminated unless great care is taken.

Milk must be kept *clean, cool and covered*. It absorbs smells rapidly, so it should never be placed near strongly smelling foods. It should be kept in a refrigerator, in spotlessly clean vessels. The *measure* should stand on a clean plate and be washed in cold running water before and after use.

Diseases which may be conveyed by milk include:

　　Tuberculosis of bones and joints
　　Diphtheria
　　Scarlet fever
　　Typhoid fever
　　Epidemic diarrhoea, especially gastroenteritis of infants
　　Tonsillitis

Milk may be infected:

　　By a diseased cow
　　During milking
　　In transit　　　　⎫ By people who carry disease-
　　At the collecting depot ⎬ bearing germs in their noses or
　　　　　　　　　　　⎭ throats, or on their hands

After delivery, especially if it is left exposed in a dirty kitchen, where flies can reach it

On a dairy farm the sheds which house the herd should be built so that they can be kept clean easily. They should be light and well ventilated. The stalls should be arranged so that excreta from the cows can be flushed away along specially constructed channels.

The cows must be healthy and free from tuberculosis. Their flanks and udders should be groomed and washed before milking commences.

Milkers should wear clean overalls and caps. Hands and nails must be washed before milking. A milker who has a sore throat or has been in contact with any infectious disease must not be allowed near the cows until given permission.

Utensils should be steam sterilized, and electric milking apparatus should be used where possible.

In transit the milk must be protected in glass-lined tanks or sealed bottles. If churns have to be used, they must be properly sterilized and covered.

Graded Milks

Graded milks are an attempt to supply cleaner milk to the public or *safe milk* as it is called.

Tuberculin tested milk is milk from cows which have been tested for tuberculosis every six months. If this milk is bottled on the farm, the words 'farm bottled' may be added.

Pasteurized milk is milk which has been cooled and filtered, then brought to a temperature of 72° C (162° F) for 15 seconds, then cooled rapidly to 50° F. This is the high temperature, short time method, most commonly used now.

Dried milk is milk which is reduced to one-eighth its bulk, all the water having been driven off by evaporation.

Condensed milk is milk which has been reduced to one-third its bulk, part of the water having been driven off, and sugar added.

Food Poisoning

Food poisoning may be the result of eating imperfectly cooked or decomposing food, or it may be due to eating contaminated or decomposing tinned food.

Two-thirds of outbreaks are caused by meat products, usually 'made-up' dishes like twice-cooked meat, pies, brawn, pressed beef, etc., and should be avoided unless home made and kept in a refrigerator until eaten. Soup should always be well boiled if it has to be heated up.

The golden rule to prevent food poisoning is to wash your hands before you handle food, and always after using the lavatory. Patients and children must have the opportunity of doing this, and the example of seeing nurses doing it.

A nurse should not handle food if she has a septic finger, or a cold.

All crockery and cutlery should be washed up in really hot soapy water and rinsed in clean water. See that drying up and dishcloths are kept clean and are boiled frequently.

Paper tissues are more hygienic than handkerchiefs, and whenever possible use paper towels for drying dishes and in place of hand towels.

6

The Health of the Nurse

In any kind of work the need for proper exercise and enjoyable recreation is recognized as being equally important with the necessity for sufficient *food*, the right kind of *clothing*, and adequate *sleep* in a restful, well ventilated atmosphere.

People who work or live for too long a period in one atmosphere tend to lose their vitality and initiative. They become stagnant in mind and body, they become easily depressed, and their physical health suffers.

In all hospitals, and especially in the world of long term illness where patients may have to be cared for until the inevitable end, the necessity for stimulating outside interests for the nursing staff cannot be too strongly emphasized.

When we remember that nursing deals with human lives, we realize that women who undertake this work should possess a clear brain, capable, gentle hands and sound common sense, and that they should form such habits and cultivate such interests as will keep them fit physically and mentally. Good and sufficient *sleep* is essential for good health. During sleep the body cells have time to repair themselves and fresh energy is built up. Circulation, digestion and respiration continue at a much slower rate. The nervous system has complete rest. The amount of sleep needed varies in individuals, but a nurse should try and obtain seven or eight hours each night.

Exercise is also necessary for a healthy body, preferably in the open air. It is far better for the nurse to have a good night's sleep every night, and to spend her daily off duty in walking, playing tennis, swimming, or the carrying on of some hobby or outside interest, than to sleep during the day.

Nurses will realize the importance of cleanliness, a term which includes the care of the *skin* by means of frequent baths, so as to keep the surface clean and the pores open and allow it to function properly.

A good *deodorant* should be used daily.

The teeth should be cleaned regularly at least twice a day. When they are in good condition they should be kept so by twice-yearly visits to the dentist.

The hands. On the skin and particularly down the ends of the nails are innumerable germs. Some of these, the *staphylococci* are the cause of *septic fingers*, *boils* and *abscesses*.

Germs enter the body through any prick, cut or scratch, and for this reason, it is particularly important that nurses should keep their nails short and their hands scrupulously clean and free from cracks. Avoid scrubbing the hands and always use a good hand cream after washing. Septic fingers should always be reported, or you may spread infection to your patients. Barrier creams should be applied whenever the hands have to be in water for any length of time. Immersion in strong disinfectants is dangerous and unnecessary.

The feet. The long distances to be traversed and hard floors of a hospital may at first be very trying to the feet. They should therefore be bathed every day, rubbed with methylated spirit and dusted lightly with talcum powder.

Stockings should be washed daily. Nylon dries rapidly and is very hard-wearing, therefore economical. A comfortable, well-fitting shoe, with a well shaped heel big enough for support, is essential.

When the feet ache, it is often helpful to sleep with a pillow under them or to raise the foot of the bed on a chair or on blocks, but if they remain persistently painful, medical advice must be sought. Simple exercises will usually remedy any tendency to flatness.

Corns should be treated by a qualified chiropodist, but the cause of the corns should be removed by wearing properly fitting shoes and stockings.

Chilblains are due to:

Poor circulation	Tight shoes
Lack of calcium	Exposure to cold and damp

They are best prevented by maintaining an effective circulation, i.e. by massage and exercise, and by wearing warm gloves and boots outdoors in cold weather.

Ingrowing toe nails should be prevented by cutting the nails straight across the top. If they have occurred, a doctor should be consulted.

The hair should be well brushed and combed night and morning, and washed regularly. It should always be washed after contact with a verminous patient.

The bowels. The inner wall of the bowel secretes a natural lubricant, mucus, which helps to keep the bowel contents moving. When this mucous membrane is stimulated unnaturally and too often by aperients, it loses its power to produce any mucus at all. It is better to cultivate a healthy mode of living, to plan regular, well-balanced meals, including in the diet an abundance of fruit and green vegetables, to drink plenty of water, and to give enough time to the matter at a regular time each day.

Clothing

Clothing should be adapted to weather and occupation. It should be loose, light in weight, non-irritating, and porous enough to allow of the evaporation of perspiration.

Wool does not conduct the heat of the body away, but holds the warm air near the skin. Its fibres consist of small, overlapping scales. It must be washed carefully, or it will become matted together and the garment will shrink, and lose its power of keeping the wearer warm. Properly cared for, it is the warmest fabric.

Cotton is a good conductor of heat. It is very durable but does not absorb much moisture.

Cellular cotton has interspaces filled with air, being woven with honeycomb weave, and so is warmer than ordinary cotton.

Linen, being a very good conductor of heat, is suitable for hot climates.

Leather and plastics are used for clothing which needs to be strong, durable, and weatherproof.

Nylon fabrics are cool, pretty and economical because they are so hard wearing. They can be rinsed through daily, dry quickly, and require no ironing. Mixtures of synthetic and natural fibres are particularly good from a hygienic point of view because they are easily washed, quickly dried, and are also absorbent and porous. Examples are wool and nylon, cotton and terylene, or linen and nylon.

Colour influences the warmth of a material only when it is worn on the outside of the body where it either absorbs or throws off the sun's rays. Thus a child's red coat is warmer than a white one, but black underwear is neither warmer nor cooler than white.

White absorbs heat *least*, so is *coolest*.

Black absorbs heat *most*, so is *hottest*.

Clothing should not cause constriction of any part of the body, nor impede movement.

Undergarments should be changed frequently and things worn during the day should not be slept in at night.

Because appearance reflects the personal character, a nurse will see that she is always neat, clean and attractive. A nurse's uniform worn well is one of the most attractive outfits you can have. If you know you look nice, you will feel self-confident, and your confidence will help your patients.

The personal bearing and attitude of the nurse make a great deal of difference to the patient and maintaining your personal standards will help you to keep your professional standards high.

Leisure

Nursing is one of the most demanding professions from an emotional point of view. Most hospitals are short of staff and hampered by old fashioned buildings and equipment, so you will generally be working in less than ideal conditions. Added to this you will be dealing, for the most part, either with people who are at some crisis point in their lives—acute illness, accident, birth, death—or with those who are burdened with long term illness. All of them need your emotional response as well as your practical techniques.

It is this very fact which makes nursing such rewarding work, but it can also cause nurses to become wrapped up in their job to the exclusion of other interests.

By all means go off duty and spend the rest of the evening telling your fellow nurses about the ghastly time you've had in the ward—but don't do it *every* day. Far too many nurses live in their uniforms not only in fact, but in their thoughts as well.

You need the point of view of someone who is not a nurse, just to keep things in proportion. You need to laugh or fume or rejoice over things that happen to people in offices and shops, in schools and canteens and banks, as well as in hospital wards. So when you are off duty get out of hospital and find some of your friends among people who are not nurses. When you return to the ward your contribution will be all the better for it.

The Patient in Hospital

7

The Nurse–Patient Relationship

We all need to feel safe and wanted if we are to thrive. This is why a baby needs its mother's love every bit as much as it needs her milk.

Twenty baby monkeys were all fed with milk in bottles. Ten were left in their cages and the bottles were tied to the bars. The others were taken out and cuddled while they were feeding. The first ten grew weaker and weaker, and finally died, but the others grew into fine, sturdy young monkeys. It is the same with human babies. A sick baby will fail to respond to treatment and may even die if this is not recognized. That is why a wise children's doctor will sometimes write on the prescription card, 'T.L.C. 20 mins. t.i.d.', which means, 'Tender loving care, 20 minutes three times a day.'

Do you remember being ill at home, as a child? Being put to bed. Having to do what you were told. Waking in the dark feeling sick and calling for your mother, and the relief when she came? The strange feeling that you were somehow being punished, because you had been put to bed, and yet at the same time your mother was being specially kind to you. Being given your favourite foods and told to 'See if you can manage just a little bit, darling'. Feeling all warm and safe and wanted—and then hearing the others playing downstairs, and feeling left out in the cold?

Did you ever call for a drink of water not because you were

thirsty, but just to have her company, or to get her away from the others for a minute? Do you remember the way you used to get them all doing what you wanted? Perhaps you sobbed, and said, 'Yes, it *does* hurt, ever so much!' Or did you put on the face of a little angel and murmur, 'If only I could die! Then I wouldn't be a nuisance any longer.'

And when you were feeling better did you try not to let them know too soon, because you wanted to go on being treated as 'special' for just a little bit longer?

What happens to us in childhood makes a deep and lasting impression on our personalities. It sets a pattern for our behaviour when we grow up—a pattern which it is hard to change —and this pattern has an influence on everything we do. So our experience of illness as children plays a big part in our attitude towards illness as adults. We are not conscious of it, but we go on behaving towards doctors and nurses as we did towards our parents—needing the same care, the same feeling of being safe and wanted, and trying to get it by whatever method experience has taught us is the most successful.

If you watch patients with this thought in mind you will see some of these patterns in the way they behave.

Some patients still feel that they are being punished, as they did when they were put to bed as children. They think of their illness as a kind of visitation. If they feel they deserve it they may become depressed and submissive, but if they think it is an unfair punishment they feel angry and resentful, and may complain bitterly about everything that is done for them. Their complaints are really a way of saying, 'Why are you punishing me? It isn't fair. I haven't done anything to deserve it.'

Others will call you every time you pass the end of the bed— to move their pillows, change the drinking water, pick up a fallen book, alter the light, shut the window, open the window, and so on. This is the grown up equivalent of 'Mummy, can I have a drink of water?' which really means, 'It's lonely up here. I feel left out. I feel scared!'

The strong silent type, who grits his teeth and says, 'You just carry on, Nurse. Never mind about me!' possibly had parents who loved to tell everyone what a brave boy he was, and so he learnt that this was the way to get their approval.

The little angel, who nearly broke her mother's heart by wanting to die so that she wouldn't be a nuisance any longer, finds she can still get a gratifying amount of attention by letting you discover that her feet are stone cold and then saying, 'Oh, but I didn't want to be a nuisance, Nurse!'

The wise nurse knows that caring for the patient's physical condition is only half of her work. She must nurse his mental attitude as well, because the two go hand in hand. Just as sick babies need the warmth and support of being cradled in the nurse's arms, so adult patients respond to treatment better when they have the support of knowing that the nurses are concerned about them as individuals. This helps them to feel safe, secure and cared for. Much of their behaviour is a way of saying, 'I feel anxious and frightened. I want you to understand this and to help me.'

The relationship between you and the patient is an important factor in his recovery. If the patient has confidence in you and knows that you care about him as a person his recovery will be that much quicker.

You should start to build up this relationship from the moment the patient is admitted to the ward (Chapter 9).

Coming into hospital, even if the patient has known in advance that he is going to be admitted, is a frightening experience. It is so easy for a busy nurse to forget this. To you the ward is a friendly place. You know everyone, you know what is likely to happen during the day, and you know what you have to do. The patient doesn't know a soul, he has no idea what is going to happen in the next half hour, and worst of all he doesn't know what he is expected to do. Not knowing what is expected of you can be a nasty feeling. It makes you feel alone, an outsider. Try to recall how you felt on the very first day you set foot in a ward, as a nurse. You probably had several other nurses with you, and perhaps one of the tutors, so it wasn't too bad. But suppose you had been quite alone. What a rush of gratitude you would have felt for the person who came up to you and said, 'Hallo! I'll show you what to do. If you want to know anything, just ask me.' This is how the patient feels.

When people are scared they don't take in what is said to them as quickly as they would normally do, so never hurry over admitting a patient if you can possibly help it. You will probably remember only too well the times when someone has said to you 'For goodness sake, Nurse! I've told you—it's there in front of your nose!'—and still you couldn't see it, because you were scared.

Don't talk to him too much, just at first, because he won't take it in, but give him a chance to talk to you if he wants to. Sit down with him and let him see that he has your full attention. This in itself will relieve his anxiety a little, and he will begin to have confidence in you.

At this stage his mind is probably as full of worries about what he has left behind him as it is of what lies ahead. This is particularly so with people who live alone, or those who may have been admitted quickly, perhaps after only a few days' illness.

He heard the ambulance man slam the front door, but he thinks the kitchen window is still open and someone might get in. He hasn't seen the milkman to tell him to stop delivery. There's some cheese in the larder, and some bacon—won't it go bad? Who will pay the rent while he's in hospital? Old people, especially, worry about who will feed the budgie or the cat. Yes, they seem unimportant problems compared with the fact that he has a large gastric ulcer—but only to you. To him they may be *more* important, and lying in bed worrying over them is the worst possible treatment for the ulcer.

Make a note of what he says and tell him that these things will be seen to. Then be sure to let sister know, so that she can get in touch with the medical social worker. When the patient hears that the social worker has taken care of everything he will feel much happier, and he will relax, because he knows he can trust you.

You can strengthen this relationship of trust and confidence, which is so important to his recovery, in the following ways:

45

1. By knowing your job.
2. By treating him as a person, not just as a 'case'.
3. By having a professional attitude towards your work.

Know Your Job

Being a bedside nurse is essentially practical work. You like using your hands to help people. This is one of your reasons for taking up nursing. So make up your mind that you will be an expert at practical nursing. No painful injections; no patients who stifle a gasp as you lift them; no fumbling catheterizations; no dropped instruments when *you* are doing the dressing; no patient who looks all of a heap after you have rearranged his pillows; no one with bedsores, or a dirty mouth, if you have anything to do with it. Take a pride in your work. Don't let anything go by which you can't understand. Ask questions. Watch how Sister and the senior nurses do it, and practise hard.

Knowing that you can do things well gives you pleasure, and confidence in yourself. It shows in your manner, and the patient knows he is in good hands when you come to him.

Treat the Patient as a Person

Imagination is one of your most useful tools. Try always to put yourself in the patient's place and understand what he is feeling. If you can do this you will realize for yourself how important it is to explain what you are going to do before you start a treatment. You will understand his need for privacy, and no one will have to remind you about drawing the curtains round his bed, or screening him in the bathroom.

It is so easy, in a ward of 20 or 30 beds, to forget that most people sleep in a bedroom all their lives, not in a dormitory. They live in places where you can lock the door when you go to the lavatory, or have a bath. If they want to strip and have a wash down they usually do it by themselves, not as one of half-a-dozen others in a row. Investigations have shown that

46

patients would rather have privacy than any amount of brightly painted ceilings, or new curtains. Don't get into the way of treating patients as if they were children in a communal bathing tent.

Try whenever you can to talk to patients, and even more important, to let them talk to you. This is just as much a part of nursing as is making a bed or doing a dressing. If you can spare a few minutes to sit down by someone's bed, or with a group of up patients, this is ideal, but in many wards you will be too busy. So while you are making his bed, or doing his dressing, talk to him as well. You already know where his home is, whether he is married, and what work he does, so you have quite a lot to go on. Remember that your purpose is to show him that you are interested in *him*. Talking about the film you saw last night, or the fun you had with your boy friend, may amuse him for a while, but don't overdo it because it doesn't give him the assurance that you are concerned about *his* welfare. Find out what his hobbies are, how the children are getting on, who is coming to see him at visiting time, has he heard from the people at work yet, and whether there is anything he is worried about.

As you move from ward to ward during your training you will find that your relationship with patients will vary slightly according to the type of ward you are in.

It usually happens that the pace of a surgical ward is quicker than that of any other. Although the patients in it will suffer some degree of shock, the mental states of these people tend to be relieved by the sense that something is being done, a definite step has been taken to alleviate their condition. They know that, unpleasant though it may be, surgery will give them a hope and probably safety.

They may even feel a bit proud of having an operation. It is something to show for being away from work, something to make a man a bit of a hero.

The best way you can help these patients is to support and comfort them through the ordeal of the operation, and then to help them become independent again as soon as possible.

In a medical, skin or orthopaedic ward, the length of illness may have had deep effects on a patient's mind. Naturally a man who has been laid off for weeks, perhaps months, and who sees no end to it, is going to be anxious and worried about many things. A woman will be longing to get back to her home and family.

Any patient with long term illness will need all you can give of patience, compassion and encouragement. Be careful never to promise wonders just to bolster them up, for they will lose their confidence in you when the promises do not come true. But do maintain a positive attitude towards them. Encourage them to do as much as they are allowed. Praise them for every step forward. Look for ways in which they can help you. People who are ill for a long time feel so useless. Thank the ones who get up and give a hand with the light tasks, and so make them feel that they are useful members of the ward family.

Children and old people have special needs, and these are dealt with in separate chapters, but there are two other groups of patients who may cause you some worry.

1. *The difficult patient*

Most patients are only too grateful for what you do for them. Many show amazing courage and a marvellous capacity for adjusting to pain or limitation. But occasionally you *will* come across one who is really unpleasant. The woman who complains, sweetly and reasonably, to sister, the doctor, matron, her relatives, and quite deliberately stirs up as much trouble for the nurses as she possibly can; the man who has a never ending store of filthy stories, and sickens every nurse who has to attend him; the foul-mouthed old person who positively enjoys upsetting his urinal the moment his sheets have been changed.

Looking after this kind of patient can be a trial for an experienced nurse, and can make life a misery for the inexperienced. Our natural response is to avoid going near him, or her, as much as we can, and even to push the job off on to another nurse if possible. But this is the worst thing we can do, for this kind of patient has a sick mental outlook as well as a sick body, and as nurses we are as much concerned with his mind as we are with his physical condition. Sometimes such a patient may benefit from psychiatric treatment, and if he thinks this is the case his doctor will ask the psychiatrist to see him, but more often the burden of coping with him falls on the nursing staff, and then it may help if you keep two points in mind.

Firstly, what this patient needs is *more* attention, not less. However hard it may be for you to believe it, behaviour like this *is* a cry for help. Somewhere, sometime, probably in childhood, this patient has been badly hurt, perhaps over a long period, and now he is trying to get his own back. No happy person deliberately hits out at others like this. Underneath the apparently malicious satisfaction is a very unhappy person indeed.

Secondly, you will find it easier to deal with this kind of patient, and less of a strain, if you make it a real team effort. Talk over the difficulties of nursing him with the other nurses, and with Sister and his doctor too, and work out a plan of campaign together. You can ask if the work can be shared out so that the junior nurses do not have to carry the bulk of it. Get into the way of looking on him as a challenge to your skill. Do your best to ignore the difficult behaviour. The less you react the less satisfying he will find it. See who can be the first to get a normal response from him, and share your successes with each other so that you can all benefit and learn how best to approach him. Perhaps the most important thing of all—do everything you can to find something on which you can genuinely compliment him. These people often feel desperately inferior beneath the surface, and this method has been known to work wonders, particularly if you can let the other patients hear the compliments as well. In fact, this patient needs what all patients need—the assurance that you care about *him*—but he needs it much more than the others, not less.

Above all, don't let him spread dissension among you by telling lies about one nurse to another, or making a favourite of one and rejecting the rest. He is a ward problem, so make his nursing a ward effort in which you all stand together.

2. *Those whose questions are hard to answer*

When patients ask questions about their progress the nurse should always refer them to sister or the doctor. 'How long shall I be in hospital?' 'Shall I have to have an operation?' 'When am I going to start walking again?' These are questions which you should not attempt to answer, unless Sister has told you what to say.

But when patients are talking to you it is sometimes difficult, and indeed unwise, to remain silent in face of a direct question, because silence in itself will be interpreted by the patient as an answer. To straightforward questions like those above you can easily say, 'I don't know, Mr Smith. I'll ask Sister to have a word with you.' But suppose the patient says, 'Shall I always be paralysed?' or, 'Do you think I'm slipping back, Nurse?' To say 'I don't know,' confirms that there is a doubt about the matter, yet to say 'Of course not!' may buoy the patient up with false hopes, and postpone the adjustment to his condition which he will inevitably have to make, sooner or later.

Perhaps the most distressing problem for a nurse to face is how to answer 'Shall I ever get better?' or even, 'Am I going to die?' There is no easy solution, but it may help if we realize that a direct answer is not the only possibility open to us.

Our wish is to help the patient. When we want to help a patient physically we don't always do what appears at first sight to be the obvious thing. For example, if a patient spills food down his pyjama jacket at meal times we don't necessarily decide that in future he must be fed. We first look at the situation and ask ourselves why he is spilling his food. Perhaps he is slumped down in bed and needs sitting up properly. Maybe he hasn't got his teeth in. It could be that for some reason he thinks he must hurry, and so gulps his food. Perhaps his hand is not steady and he can't manage soup, or custard, or a soft boiled egg. There may be many reasons, and if the help we give is to be effective we must discover where the difficulty lies.

In the same way patients may have a number of reasons for asking, 'Am I going to die?' or, 'Shall I ever get better?' Instead of a direct answer, or an equally informative silence, try saying, 'What makes you say that, Mr Smith?' You may find he has overheard something and has misunderstood what was meant; or his wife said there was a programme on television and they said it was incurable; or he thinks the chap in the bed by the door had the same thing, and he's gone, hasn't he? Or perhaps he is quite aware that his condition is serious and there are business or family affairs he wants to see to, while he is still capable of doing so. Whatever it is you will get some indication of his thoughts by his reply to *your* question. You can then quite naturally say, 'I think Sister can help you with this, Mr Smith. I'll ask her to come and talk to you,' and when you tell sister about it she will be in a better position to help him if she knows in advance a little of what is in his mind.

Have a Professional Attitude

Having a professional attitude means regarding your work primarily as a way of giving service to other people. Not that it isn't right that you should have a higher salary, and shorter hours, and better conditions, but that even more than these things you really want to do a job in which you help people. In nursing it simply means that in every situation you put the welfare of the patients first.

You may feel like saying, 'Yes, of course! We all do that.' But have you really thought out the implications? It means such ordinary things as being punctual; seeing that your uniform is always clean, because a dirty uniform increases cross infection, so do dirty hair and dirty nails. When you are rushed for time, and no one is looking, being professional means that you are still as meticulous over your techniques as you would be if sister were watching. You give as much attention to the difficult patients as you do the charming ones. Although you know the boy in the corner has fallen for you, and you like him a lot, you treat it lightly, because you know he is seeing you with a halo round your head, and you may both feel differently when he has been discharged a few weeks. It means that although you have a happy relationship with the patients, and talk to them as much as you can, you learn to leave your own problems on the other side of the ward door and not to unload them on the patients. Being human you sometimes disagree with other people, or feel moody and irritable, but because you are also a professional you don't explode in the middle of the ward. You wait until you are in the staff room, and have it out with them then.

The professional person understands that she is working as a member of a team, and she shows by her behaviour towards them that she respects the contribution made by the other members. In the hospital team there are nurses, doctors, domestic staff, clerks, engineers, porters, cooks, and many others, all of whom are working in some way towards the patient's recovery, and you should treat all of them with the courtesy you expect for yourself.

Patients see far more than nurses think they do, and you might be surprised to know how accurately they can sum you up. One of the things they are quick to notice is the way a nurse behaves towards other members of the staff, and the nurse who is sarcastic to her juniors or rude to non-nursing staff soon loses their respect.

You cannot *demand* a patient's trust, but if you know your job, are genuinely interested in him, and show that you are a professional person, he will freely give it to you. Once you have experienced the value, and the satisfaction, of a good nurse–patient relationship, you will want to use it with just as much skill as you use your practical techniques, and you will understand how necessary it is to study this aspect of your work.

8

Beds and Bed-making

Bed-making is the first thing the new nurse learns to do, and it is one of the most important of all her nursing duties. The bed is the patient's home for a good part of his stay. His comfort, rest and sleep depend very much on the nurse's skill and efficiency. Like all skills, perfection only comes by practice, first in the classroom, and then in the wards.

It need never be a boring task. This is the time to get to know your patients, to talk to them and let them talk to you. His grateful 'Oh, Nurse, I'm so glad you've come, it is wonderful to have my bed made,' will be your reward.

However, if a patient is unconscious, or too ill to appear to be listening, *never* discuss his condition, treatment, or operation with another nurse anywhere near him. You do not know how much may penetrate to his mind and be remembered.

To Make an Occupied Bed

Take to the bedside a trolley with clean linen, the equipment for treating the patient's pressure areas and a receptacle for soiled linen.

Exclude draughts by closing nearby windows. Draw the bed curtains and place a bed stripper, or two chairs back to back, at the foot of the bed.

If the patient is *allowed to get up* for bed-making:

Help him to put on his dressing-gown and slippers and seat him in a comfortable chair at the side of the bed where you can see him. Make sure that he is warm and if necessary wrap a blanket round him. While you are making the bed keep a careful eye on him, so that you will notice at once if the effort of sitting out of bed is too much for him.

If the patient may not get out of bed, but is *allowed to lie down flat*:

Starting at the head of the bed, untuck the bedclothes down to the foot.

Remove each article separately, folding it loosely and hanging it over the backs of the chairs with the lower end turned under and resting on the seat of a chair. Make certain that no part of the bedclothes trails on the floor, because this is one of the ways in which germs are spread.

Leave the last blanket on as a cover for the patient and remove the top sheet by drawing it down towards the foot of the bed, underneath the blanket.

Take out all the pillows except one and lay the patient flat.

See which side of the bed has the least amount of drawsheet tucked in.

The nurse on this side leans over the patient, keeping him covered with the blanket, places one forearm behind his shoulders and the other under his buttocks, and gently rolls him over towards her, supporting him in this position while the other nurse moves the pillow so that his head is resting comfortably.

Straighten the underblanket and sheet, brushing out any crumbs and tucking the sheet in firmly.

Tuck in about twelve inches of the drawsheet and gather the rest in a roll against the patient's back.

Roll the patient gently on to his back and right over to the other side, keeping him covered and supported and moving the pillow so that he is comfortable.

Brush and straighten out the sheet and underblanket on the other side and tuck them in.

Unroll the drawsheet, brush it free of crumbs and tuck it in firmly, folding the extra length under the mattress, so that the patient has a cool, fresh portion on which to lie.

If necessary attend to the patient's pressure areas at this stage.

Then roll him gently on to his back again, putting his pillows back and arranging them comfortably with their open ends away from the ward door.

Spread the top sheet over the bed and withdraw the blanket covering the patient.

Tuck the sheet in at the bottom, envelope fashion, making a good pleat over his feet so that he can move without restriction.

Replace each blanket separately, pleating each one over his feet and making sure that they come high enough up the bed to cover his shoulders.

Replace the counterpane. Do not pleat it over the feet, but leave the sides hanging loose with mitred corners.

Turn down the top sheet.

If the patient *must sit upright*:
Strip the top bedclothes, leaving one blanket covering the patient.

Untuck the bottom sheet, lift the patient's feet, brush out the crumbs, straighten the underblanket and tuck the sheet in again firmly.

Keeping the patient well covered, lift him down to the bottom of the bed.

One nurse now supports him while the other remakes the top part of the bed.

Lift the patient back and finish the rest of the bed.

If the patient may not be moved in this way two nurses must lift him where he is, while a third straightens the underblanket, tucks in the sheet and pulls the drawsheet through.

Again, if necessary, attend to his pressure areas at this stage.

TO CHANGE THE BOTTOM SHEET

If the patient *may lie down*:
Roll the clean sheet lengthwise.

Strip the top of the bed and roll the patient to one side, keeping him covered with the blanket.

Untuck the drawsheet and the bottom sheet.

Roll the bottom sheet up against the patient's back, together with the drawsheet and plastic sheeting.

Place the clean sheet in position, tucking it in firmly all along the side and rolling the surplus up against the patient's back.

Unroll the drawsheet and plastic sheeting and tuck in about twelve inches of the drawsheet.

Roll the patient over to the other side, take out the soiled sheet, unroll the clean one and the drawsheet, and complete the bed in the usual way.

If the patient *may sit up*:

Roll the sheet widthways and put it in from the head of the bed.

Lift the patient down to the bottom of the bed and support him.

Remove the drawsheet and plastic sheeting.

Untuck the bottom sheet from the head of the bed and roll it down as far as possible. Tuck the clean sheet in and roll it down to meet the soiled one.

Replace the drawsheet and plastic sheeting.

Lift the patient back again, pull the soiled sheet out, roll the clean one down and tuck it in. Be careful to keep the patient covered and supported all the time.

If the patient must not be moved to the foot of the bed three nurses will be needed—two to raise him while the third rolls the sheets down and replaces the drawsheet and plastic sheeting.

SOILED AND FOUL LINEN

After bed-making *soiled linen* is placed in the soiled linen container, sealed, and sent to the laundry.

Foul linen, that is, linen soiled with urine or faeces, should be placed in a special foul linen container, sealed, and sent to the laundry at the earliest possible moment.

Soiled and foul linen contains innumerable germs. It should

never be shaken about, counted in the ward, or handled more than is absolutely necessary, and nurses should always wash their hands after touching it.

DOs AND DON'Ts

Some nurses get into the habit of patting the bed as they make it. They shake the pillows up and arrange them in position, then give them a final pat, just as the patient leans back on them. They pull the bedclothes comfortably around his shoulders, then pat them—and him. They tuck the sides in firmly, then pat the top bedclothes down. They mitre the corners of the counterpane, and give a final satisfied pat—right against the patient's feet.

After one or two bed-making sessions the patient knows what is coming and waits in irritated anticipation for each pat.

This is something you can easily observe in other nurses, but you will never notice it in yourself. The best thing to do is to ask your partner to watch you, and to pull you up every time you do it. Don't be a patter!

When you have finished making the bed always ask the patient if he is comfortable before leaving him. See that his head is properly supported, that the clothes are not tight over his chest and feet, and that his locker is by his side with everything he needs within reach.

Special Beds

Operation bed. This is made up in the ordinary way as far as the drawsheet.

Spread the top sheet, the blankets and the counterpane on the bed, but do not tuck them in.

Fold the top sheet down in the ordinary way.

Fold back the sheet and blankets at the foot of the bed, and turn the counterpane under, so that the folds are flush with the end of the mattress.

Turn the sides of the bedclothes up and on to the top of the bed in one piece.

Fold the clothes up from the bottom of the bed, and down from the top, making a pack which is easy to remove and to replace when the patient is put in the bed.

Remove all pillows and place them on a chair beside the bed.

Place a small plastic sheet and towel at the head of the bed in case the patient vomits.

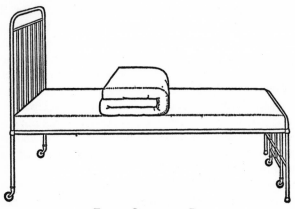

FIG. 4. OPERATION BED

The following articles will have been taken to theatre by the nurse who went with the patient, and will be brought back by her when she returns with him to the ward:

Vomit bowl with dressing towel
Sponge holder with gauze swab in position
Mouth gag
Tongue depressor
Tongue forceps
In addition the following articles should be ready on his locker:
Bowl of wool swabs in water
Bowl of dry gauze swabs
Forceps for removing swabs from sponge holder
Receiver or disposal bag for airway and forceps
Receiver or disposal bag for swabs.

Beds and Bed-making

Emergency or accident bed

This is prepared in the same way as an operation bed, but a plastic sheet and an admission blanket are used to protect the bottom bedclothes and another admission blanket is placed ready to cover the patient. The bedclothes are made into a pack and placed over an electric pad or hot bottles, and, if necessary, fracture boards are placed under the mattress to make the bed level and firm.

Fracture bed

Place fracture boards under the mattress to prevent it from sagging and, if an extension is to be applied to a limb, have blocks ready to raise the foot of the bed so as to prevent the patient's body from being pulled down the bed.

Divided bed

This is used when traction is applied to the lower limb, and occasionally when a leg has been amputated.

Place a sheet with a folded blanket inside it over the upper part of the patient's body. Lay another sheet on the lower half of the bed and tuck it in the bottom. On this lay a folded blanket and turn the sheet over it. The lower half of the bedclothes should overlap the upper half for a few inches.

Plaster bed

Place fracture boards under the mattress. Lay the limb which has been encased in plaster of Paris on waterproof sheeting and a drawsheet to protect the bedclothes. Cover the limb with a cradle. Do not apply hot water bottles unless specially ordered to do so by the doctor. The plaster may become too hot and cause a burn.

Turn back the lower half of the bedclothes and expose the part to the air until it is dry. Keep the other limb warm by means of a long woollen stocking and a blanket. The toes of the foot which is exposed may be kept warm by means of a toe-cap made of gauze tissue or a rolled up bedsock.

When the plaster is dry, remove the waterproof sheeting and drawsheet, place the limb on a pillow and make up the bed in the ordinary way.

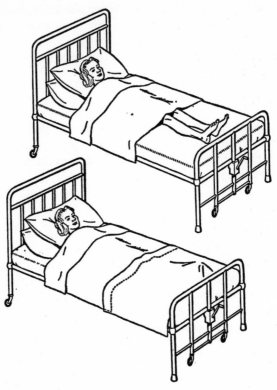

FIG. 5. A DIVIDED BED   *Above*: THE FIRST STAGE   *Below*: COMPLETED

Amputation bed

The end of the stump is kept in position by means of a cloth and sandbags.

A cradle must be used to take the weight of the bedclothes. A divided bed is sometimes used, but many surgeons prefer the bed to be made in the ordinary way.

Bed for a breathless patient

Some patients with disease of the lungs or heart find breathing difficult. They can be helped by supporting them in a sitting position with plenty of pillows and a backrest.

Sometimes a bed-table with a small pillow on it for the patient to lean on is helpful.

Pressure is relieved by air rings or pads and a cradle may also be needed.

To prevent the patient slipping down in the bed the foot of the bed may be raised on low blocks, or a padded board may be provided against which his feet can rest. Pillows should not be placed under the knees for this purpose because the pressure, and the inability of the patient to move his legs, may cause thrombosis (the formation of blood clots in the veins).

Ripple beds

Ripple beds should be used for all heavy patients and for those who are liable to develop bed sores. They are special thin tubular air mattresses which are placed on top of the ordinary ones. An electrically controlled pump causes continuous slight movement which gently massages the parts of the body lying on it, and so stimulates the circulation and relieves pressure at the same time.

Positions Used in Nursing

Recumbent. The patient is placed flat in bed with one pillow under the head. This position is used for patients who must have complete rest, e.g. acute heart case; acute rheumatism; shock.

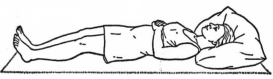

FIG. 6. THE RECUMBENT POSITION

Semi-recumbent. The patient is half propped up with several pillows or a reclining bedrest. The usual position in convalescence.

Left lateral. The patient lies on her left side with her buttocks on the edge of the bed and her thighs and knees flexed, used when giving an enema or doing a rectal examination.

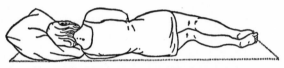

FIG. 7. THE LEFT LATERAL POSITION

Sims's position. This is an exaggeration of the left lateral position. It is a more prone attitude with the chest and head resting on a low pillow and the left arm lying behind the back to allow a good view of the vulva. Used for vaginal examinations.

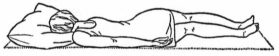

FIG. 8. SIMS'S POSITION

Fowler's position. The patient is propped upright in a sitting position.

Fowler's position assists breathing as there is less pressure on the diaphragm and so chest and lung complications are prevented. It is more comfortable after chest operations and after amputations of the breast.

It is also valuable for its psychological effect, as a patient who can sit up and see what is going on around him feels better than one who has to lie flat.

Semi-prone position. This is the safest position for an unconscious patient. He is placed on his side with his upper leg and arm bent at right-angles. His lower arm is gently drawn from under his body until it lies on the bed behind him.

His head is turned to the side and his neck slightly extended. He does *not* have a pillow under his head.

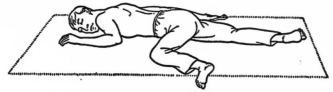

FIG. 9. THE SEMI-PRONE POSITION

In this position his tongue cannot fall back and block his airway and any vomit or blood will drain out of his mouth instead of being breathed into his lungs.

Hot Water Bottles

Rubber hot water bottles should be three-quarters filled with hot, not boiling water. Metal and stone bottles should not be used except in emergency when there is nothing else. If they are used they should be warmed first in order to prevent cracking or sudden expansion of the metal, then filled to capacity.

The washer and screw top must be tested each time a bottle is used.

In the case of rubber bottles, expel the air and in all cases make sure the bottle does not leak.

Use a funnel when filling. Cover all hot water bottles with a thick bag and tie securely. Place the bottle on top of the blanket in such a way that it cannot roll over and rest against the patient.

Children, restless patients, unconscious patients, old people and paralysed people, and patients recovering from an anaesthetic are particularly liable to receive hot water bottle burns, and hot bottles should never be left in their beds. The bed should be well warmed before the patient is put into it, and then all bottles should be removed.

In a cot, the bottle should be placed under the mattress with the neck end towards the foot of the cot.

Severe burns may be suffered by the patient touching a hot bottle when insufficient care has been taken to see that it is suitably placed and protected. This has always been regarded as being a nursing disgrace.

N.B.—Hot water bottles are *never* used with electric cradles or electric blankets because, should they leak, there is a danger of electrocution.

Lifting Patients

It is most important that you should learn to lift patients correctly, both for the patients' sake and for your own.

Most people bend over from the waist when picking up something heavy, and keep their legs almost straight. Watch a man digging in his garden, or a woman picking up a child. This way leads straight to troubles like backache or rupture, because it puts the full strain on the muscles of the back and abdomen.

If, on the other hand, you keep your back straight and bend your knees it is possible to lift really heavy weights with no ill effects at all because this method puts the strain on the leg muscles, which are far stronger than those of the back.

There are two methods which are widely used by nurses when lifting patients. These are the 'orthodox lift' and the 'shoulder lift'. They are explained by the illustrations in the Plates section and you should practise them until they are second nature to you. The essence of each of them is to *keep your back straight* and *bend your knees*.

9

Admitting Patients and Giving Routine Care

Going into hospital is a frightening thing for most people. To a nurse the hospital smell—a mixture of disinfectant, floor polish and stew—goes almost unnoticed, she is so used to it, but to the new patient being escorted down the endless corridors it opens up a whole new world of anxiety, and the glimpses he gets of strange equipment and people on stretchers do nothing to lessen his apprehension.

People coming into hospital are afraid. They are afraid of pain; of having embarrassing things done to them; of being cut off from home; of making a fool of themselves; of being a nuisance; of not being told anything.

You may feel this is too long a list to cope with in the middle of a busy day, but try to remember the last fear—of not being told anything. How often have people come out of hospital and said to their friends, 'Of course, they never tell you anything!' If you can deal with this fear you will go a long way towards removing the others.

Welcoming the Patient

Start by telling the patient your name. Greet him and his relatives with a smile. Many nurses are so wrapped up in their work that they hardly ever smile, yet it is one of the quickest ways of reassuring people.

Find somewhere where they can sit down while you fill in the admission forms. In some hospitals admission forms are filled in at the reception centre before the patient comes to the ward, but if you are completing them in the ward you will need to take down the following information:

Date	Religion
Name and address of patient	Age
Whether married or single	Occupation
Name and address of private doctor	
Name of physician or surgeon in charge of the patient	
Name, address and telephone number of next of kin	

If the patient's next of kin is not on the telephone be sure to get the name, address and telephone number of a relative, friend or neighbour who would be willing to take a message.

It is common practice now to place an identification band round the new patient's wrist, on which will be written his own name, that of his doctor, any special information, and a serial number. You will be informed of this procedure in each ward.

If the patient is likely to need an *operation*, his consent, or in the case of a child, that of the nearest relative, must be obtained. In cases of dangerous illness, the patient must be placed on the *free visiting list*, and the relatives informed that they can visit him at any time.

When you have finished take the patient to his bed and tell his relatives that they will be able to see him again to say goodbye.

Introduce him to the patients in the beds on either side of him.

If he is allowed to get up tell him where the lavatory is. Don't just nod towards the end of the ward. All doors look alike to a new patient. Tell him plainly that it's through the swing door and then the third on the left—or whatever.

If he is not to get up tell him what to ask for. 'Urinal', 'bottle', 'bedpan', 'commode', are everyday words to a nurse, but to many a patient they are a new and embarrassing language.

Give him a brief outline of the ward routine, the meal times, when the doctors do their rounds, the visiting hours and the time the night staff come on duty.

Help him to put his things in his locker and see that he is comfortably settled in bed. Make sure that he is warm enough. Anxious people often have cold feet, even in summer. When you have done all that you can, tell him that you will be about in the ward and if there is anything he wants you will be glad to help him. Try to keep a special eye on him for the rest of the day, remembering how lost he may be feeling—and don't forget that friendly smile.

Spiritual care. A priest of each denomination will visit any patients who belong to his Church from time to time. If any patient wishes to see his minister the nurse informs the matron's office so that the clergyman in question may be informed.

Whenever a patient is visited by a clergyman, the nurse must draw the curtains around his bed and see that the ward is kept as quiet as possible.

Routine procedure on the admission of a patient

Take the patient's temperature, pulse and respiration, noting his general condition and symptoms and reporting them to the person in charge of the ward.

Unless there are contra-indications, e.g. a raised temperature or feebleness, etc., offer the patient a bath and take this opportunity of noting and reporting any sores, bruises, rashes or other abnormalities. As soon as possible get a specimen of urine for testing (p. 113).

Each hospital has its own special procedure with regard to a patient's clothing and valuables. As a rule he keeps by him only the minimum of his possessions, but if the relatives cannot take his clothes and valuables home, the nurse must obtain instructions with regard to them from the sister or nurse in charge of the ward.

Transfer and Discharge of Patients

When a patient is transferred to another hospital, the nurse in charge must see that his relatives are notified and that all his possessions are sent with him, together with particulars of his medical history, X-ray films and records of any special examinations and treatments he may have had.

It is especially important to see that the patient's body and head are absolutely clean.

On discharge, clothing and any personal possessions are returned to the patient and he is informed if and when he is required to attend the Out Patient Department for treatment. A note will be sent to his private doctor. If he has a wound which needs dressing give him enough wool, gauze, etc. to enable the district nurse to attend to him adequately until his own doctor can call and prescribe a fresh supply. See that he has any medicine or tablets that he should be taking, and that he understands the dosage. His relatives must be told of his discharge in good time, so that they can come and fetch him. If this is not possible a car and driver will be supplied to take him home. The nurse must see that the patient is ready at the correct time, so that busy people are not kept waiting.

Points to Note Before Carrying Out Any Nursing Procedure

Before carrying out any treatment whatsoever to a patient, or before getting him ready for sister or the doctor for any examination or procedure, there are certain rules to be observed. To save space, they will not be repeated at the beginning of each little section of your book. Once you know them you will do them as routine.

1. Always tell the patient what you are going to do. If the trolley you are putting by the bedside is for the doctor, you can simply say, 'Your doctor is coming to have a look at you, and these are a few things he may want.' Do not leave the patient frightened, wondering what is going to happen.

2. Close any near-by windows and draw the curtains round the bed to ensure privacy. Remember that what is familiar to you may be very embarrassing for a patient.

3. Provide a good light.

4. Arrange the bedclothes so as to expose the patient as little as possible, while leaving a good view of the part to be examined.

5. Make sure that the patient is perfectly clean.

6. If the patient is a woman, remain with her throughout any examination.

7. After treatment, leave the patient comfortable. Tidy up, but leave at hand necessary articles for use in an emergency.

8. In all cases where a patient needs to sit up in bed for treatment, see that he wears a shoulder blanket or bedjacket.

9. Before any internal examination see that the bowels and bladder are empty.

10. When everything is finished, clear away and wash or sterilize the articles used. Leave the patient warm and comfortable.

The Hygiene of the Patient

This includes the care of the patient's

Clothing	Hair
Skin	Teeth
Nails	Back
Mouth	

and the keeping of all openings of the body clean.

CLOTHING

The clothing must always be changed when necessary and should be loose, comfortable and convenient. If rest is essential for the patient, the garments should be open at the back so as to slip easily on and off.

Unless very ill, let the patient wear his own garments, in which he will feel more at ease.

CARE OF THE SKIN

Since the function of the skin is to remove waste and to help to regulate the temperature of the body, it should be kept clean by frequent bathing. In her work of caring for the sick a nurse should attend to the toilet, and every detail affecting the patient's well-being, in such a way as to spare him any embarrassment.

A patient should be washed twice a day and, owing to the great risk of infection being carried to the mouth and spreading through the body, the hands should always be washed after the patient has used a bedpan or been to the lavatory.

If possible a bath should be given daily, but never less than once a week. When a bath is not given, the patient's groins and buttocks must be washed at least once a day.

The temperature of the water for a tepid bath is about 32° C (90° F) cooling to about 27° C (80·6° F) and of a hot bath it is about 40·5° C (105° F.).

The nurse must always prepare the water for a patient's bath and *test* it with a *bath thermometer*. She must see that everything he requires is in readiness, e.g. soap, towels and clean clothing.

The windows must be closed and the patient must not be left alone in the bath. The door is not locked and the nurse must be within call. A screen can be placed round the bath to ensure privacy. The hot tap should be guarded so that the patient cannot touch it.

After bathing, she should see that the patient's body is clean and she should inspect the finger and toe nails and cut them if necessary.

Abnormalities, e.g. bruises, spots, cuts, deformities, etc., must be noted and reported at once to the Sister in charge of the ward.

After use, the bath is scrubbed out and disinfected with the disinfectant in general use at the hospital, and the bottle put away in a safe place afterwards. The windows must be thrown open and the bathroom left tidy and ready for use by the next patient.

BATHING A PATIENT IN BED

A patient whose temperature is higher than 37·2° C (99° F) or who is too ill to go to the bathroom is bathed in bed. Two nurses will be needed if the patient is very ill or unable to move.

To give a blanket bath

Protect the patient from draughts by closing near-by windows.
Draw the curtains round his bed.
Prepare everything likely to be used beforehand.
See that the room is warm.
Offer him a bedpan.
Put the patient's clothes to warm, and if he is allowed a hot water bottle, refill it and put it to his feet before starting to bath him.
Prepare a trolley containing the following:
Top shelf
    Two towels (one face, one body)
    Face and body flannels
    Soap and nail brush   } From patient's own locker
    Brush and comb
    Toothbrush and toothpaste
    Bowl of water at 43° C (110° F)
    Tooth mug and bowl
    Scissors and nail clippers in a receiver
    Bath thermometer
    Equipment for treating pressure areas
Lower shelf
    Clean linen
    Bath blankets from patient's locker
    Soiled linen container
    If there is no sink at hand a jug of hot water, 50° C, and a
        pail for used water will also be needed

N.B. Individual bath blankets should be used for each patient and kept in his locker. Where it is not possible to supply individual bath blankets it is better to use the top blanket from the patient's own bed and a large towel underneath him. On no account should the same bath blankets be used for several patients. This is another way in which germs are quickly spread around the ward.

Method. Remove the upper bedclothes and cover the patient with a warm blanket.

Roll the second bath blanket underneath him.

Remove the gown or pyjamas gently.

Wash and dry the face and neck thoroughly, then the arms and hands keeping the rest of the body covered. The chest and the legs and feet are then dealt with. If possible, the patient should be allowed to dip his hands and feet in the bowl of water.

A nurse must pay particular attention to the armpits, to the folds of the skin under the breasts, and to the umbilicus.

If the patient is able to do so, he is allowed, under cover of the blanket, to wash the groins and the genital organs; if he is helpless, the nurse must do it for him.

Change the water.

Roll the patient over and wash the back and buttocks.

Keep the water really hot all the time. Only uncover the part you are actually washing, and make certain that you get him dry.

Don't try to be too gentle over the actual drying. Nothing is worse than being dabbed at for minutes on end while the moisture slowly evaporates, leaving one chilled and uncomfortable.

Get a good grip on the towel, support the patient's limb firmly, and rub vigorously as you would rub yourself. So long as you take care not to hurt the patient this kind of treatment will help him to relax, and a blanket bath will be something he looks forward to, instead of a depressing procedure which he is glad to get over.

All pressure areas must be treated in the course of the bathing.

The nails should be trimmed carefully, cutting off only a little at a time, to the shape of the finger tips and cutting the toe nails straight across in order to prevent the development of ingrowing toe nails.

Roll out the bath blanket.

Put on the clean pyjamas or nightdress.
Attend to the mouth and hair.
Replace the upper bedclothes.
Give a hot drink if the patient would like one, then clear everything away and leave him (or her) tidy and comfortable.

CARE OF THE MOUTH

A patient who is able to do so should clean his teeth twice a day. Artificial teeth must be removed regularly, scrubbed and rinsed in cold water. Helpless patients and patients on a fluid diet need especial care or the teeth will decay, a bad taste will affect the appetite; sore throat and swollen glands may occur and septic absorption may make the patient very ill.

During the acute stage of an illness, the mouth should be cleaned before feeds and a drink of water given afterwards.

Articles needed on a mouth tray

1. Gallipot with warm bicarbonate of soda solution (1 teaspoonful to 1 pint) for dissolving mucus.
2. Gallipot with glycerin and borax for softening the hard dry crusts.
3. Gallipot with diluted lemon juice, when obtainable, to encourage the flow of saliva, or weak antiseptic, e.g. Glyco-Thymoline, to use for a final swabbing and so leave a pleasant taste in the mouth.
4. Jar with at least two pairs of forceps, one to hold the swabs and one to remove them. A pair of forceps that will grip, such as artery forceps, should be used, *never* pointed ones. *N.B.* A nurse must *never* use her fingers when swabbing a mouth.
5. Bowl of swabs.
6. Fine wooden sticks for cleaning between teeth.
7. Receiver or disposal bag for used swabs.
8. White petroleum jelly for cracked lips.
9. Mouth gag and tongue depressor for unconscious patient.

73

The forceps must be boiled every time they are used, otherwise infection may spread from one patient to another.

Method. Using each lotion in turn, and working from side to side, clean the lips and teeth, inside and outside, and the tongue and roof of the mouth, frequently changing the swabs. Finish by smoothing a little petroleum jelly over the lips.

If well enough, the patient can clean his own teeth with his ordinary brush and toothpaste. Finish by giving a pleasant mouthwash.

Cleaning the mouth is an important nursing procedure, because infection can start so easily in a dirty mouth and track down to the stomach and lungs, leading to serious complications.

It is also important for the patient's comfort. You know what your own mouth feels like if you have a hangover and haven't cleaned your teeth. A mouth full of sticky, half-dried mucus, with coated teeth and cracked lips, is ten times worse than this. The comfort you can bring by thorough cleaning is quite out of proportion to the effort involved, and the more frequently you do it the easier it will be.

CARE OF THE HAIR

The hair of all patients whose condition will permit of it should be washed occasionally if they have to stay in for a long time. It may be possible for a trained hairdresser to visit the wards and do this, with the help of a nurse. Arrange the patient in the position which distresses him least, e.g. a patient with difficult breathing must never be made to lie down. The bowl must be placed on a bed table in a convenient position.

In other cases, a space must be made for the bowl by:
1. Bringing the patient to the edge of the bed and placing the bowl on a chair.
2. Folding in the top of the mattress, or
3. Pulling down the mattress over the bedrail at the bottom, and placing the bowl on the wire mattress.

74

Articles needed for washing the hair in bed

Blanket, cape and towel
Towels for the hair and eyes
Wool for the ears
Bed table if necessary
Mackintosh and drawsheet to protect the bed
Washing bowl
Jugs of hot and cold water
Bath thermometer in jug
Soap solution or shampoo
Pail
Two rubber hot water bottles in covers, to help drying if the
    hair is long
Method. Slip the gown off the shoulders.
Protect the patient's shoulders with the blanket and cape.
Lightly place some cotton wool in the ears.
Give the patient a face towel to protect his eyes.
Arrange a space for the bowl to be placed under the patient's
head. Prepare the shampoo at $37 \cdot 5°$ C ($99 \cdot 5°$ F).
Rub the shampoo into the scalp with the tips of the fingers.
Rinse by pouring warm water over the head.
Repeat the shampooing process and rinse again, very
thoroughly, emptying the water into the bucket when necessary.
Remove the bowl and thoroughly dry the scalp and hair with
a warm towel.
Brush and comb gently.
Replace the mattress and pillow and arrange the ends over a
towel under which the hot water bottles have been placed, to
finish drying.

VERMINOUS PATIENTS

A nurse admitting a verminous patient should wear a closely
fitting theatre cap over her hair and an overall which completely
covers her uniform.
The patient's clothes should be tied up in a sheet and sent,

along with the bath blankets and the overall and cap worn by the nurse, to be disinfected by steam under pressure in an apparatus specially designed for the purpose.

The hairy parts of the patient's body should be shaved and the parts, after he has been bathed, smeared with white precipitate ointment.

Suleo Hair Emulsion is effective for treating verminous heads. The solution is applied to the scalp with a pipette, a small area being treated at a time until the whole head has been thoroughly covered. Wash the hair after 24 hours and then comb it daily with a fine-tooth comb until no more nits are found.

Cleaning a verminous patient is a thoroughly unpleasant task, but try to remember that, even if he does not show it, the patient is probably embarrassed that you should have to do this for him. Give him as much privacy as you can, and try not to let the other patients know about his condition.

HELPLESS AND INCONTINENT PATIENTS

Helpless and incontinent patients, on account of their lowered vitality, need to be nursed in a warm atmosphere and the ward and its outlook should be quiet and pleasant.

Where possible, helpless patients should be propped up during the day so that they can see what is going on about them, and in order to prevent congestion at the base of the lungs. Bedclothes must be warm and light in weight and cradles must be used where necessary to prevent pressure on the limbs and body.

To prevent foot drop, which may occur through weakness of the ankle, a sandbag or firm pillow may be used to support the foot, or, in some cases, a suitable splint may be applied.

The wrist also may need support on a light cock-up splint. This will be removed daily for washing and exercises.

BEDSORES

Except in rare cases, bedsores are due to want of care in nursing. Special attention should be paid to the pressure areas of all bed-ridden patients, especially those suffering from:

1. Incontinence, when the skin is often wet.
2. Paralysis, when the patient cannot move from the position in which he is lying.
3. Oedema, when the patient is not only extra heavy, but the skin is unhealthy from the lack of natural circulation.
4. Loss of weight, when the bones are just under the skin.
5. Overweight, when pressure is unusually great.

These pressure areas include the lower part of the back, the elbows, shoulder blades, heels, hips or anywhere that pressure can be seen to lie owing to the position of the patient.

Causes of bedsores are:

1. Pressure, particularly that of lying too long in one position.
2. Moisture, through insufficient care in drying and through moisture collecting in the folds of the skin of fat patients.
3. Friction (rubbing), through crumbs in the bed and creases in the sheets.
4. Pressure of splints, plasters or other apparatus.

The first symptoms of a bedsore are heat and discomfort. There will be redness and, if the pressure on the part is not relieved, the skin will crack and soon a sore will form, which can get deeper and bigger until a lot of the flesh is eaten away. Such a sore is one of the most difficult wounds to heal.

To prevent bedsores

1. Keep the parts scrupulously clean and quite dry.
2. Change the position as often as possible.
3. Attend to all the pressure areas.
4. Relieve pressure by such means as:
     A sponge or ripple bed
     Air rings
     Ring pads, i.e. tow or wool wrapped round with a bandage
     Extra pillows

5. Never use patched, darned, or rough places in a drawsheet immediately under the back.
6. Never let a patient lie in a wet bed.

Relief of pressure is vitally important for the prevention of bedsores. This is best achieved either by the use of a ripple bed, or by turning the patient every two hours.

For attending to all pressure areas, prepare a trolley containing the following articles:

Top shelf
    Bath towel   Bowl of water
    Soap in dish   Powder in sifter
    Tow   Ointment, such as Silicone or other
    Receiver for used tow   barrier cream

Lower shelf
    Two large jugs, one containing hot and the other cold water
    Pail for dirty water
    Clean sheets
    Receptacle for soiled sheets

Method of attending to a patient's back

Draw the curtains round the bed and explain to the patient what is to be done.

Remove the upper bedclothes, covering the patient with a blanket, and place a towel alongside him to avoid damping the bedclothes.

Wash and dry the back.

Lather the hand, then with a circular and kneading movement, which serves to promote circulation in the part, rub the skin thoroughly but gently and rinse and dry carefully.

A little powder may be used to complete the drying of the skin, but if the patient is incontinent, use a barrier cream instead of powder as this forms a waterproof covering for the skin.

Many hospitals now consider that massaging with soap removes the protective oils in the skin and so renders it more liable to break down. Massaging with a little powder, or with a few

78

drops of olive oil as a lubricant, are considered to be better methods.

Curtains should always be drawn round the bed before a bedpan is given. Bedpans should be warmed before use and brought to the bedside covered with a disposable cover.

Any knee pillows or air rings are removed.

The nurse helps the patient to raise himself by placing her left hand under the lower part of his body, telling him to draw his knees up while she slips the bedpan underneath the buttocks. A pad of wool may be placed on the edge of the bedpan if the patient is thin or helpless. Arrange his pillows to support him and see that his back and shoulders are warmly covered. Leave the patient alone until he is ready for help.

Remove the bedpan in the same way as it was inserted, and clean the parts thoroughly, leaving the patient dry and comfortable.

A patient who is able to attend to himself should be allowed to do so. He must wash his hands afterwards. See that a woman who is having a menstrual period is provided with a clean sanitary towel. Remove soiled ones in disposable bags. Remember that a woman can pass urine *and* faeces into a bedpan, but a man needs a urinal with a bedpan.

Bedpans and urinals should be emptied and cleaned immediately unless the contents are to be saved for inspection. The disposable type will be put straight into the incinerator. The room must be thoroughly aired but care must be taken that the patient does not contract a chill.

Nurses should always wash their hands after giving bedpans, urinals, etc.

10

Observing and Reporting

TEMPERATURE, PULSE AND RESPIRATION

Here in Britain we have, until recently, been used to having only the Fahrenheit scale for temperature. We are gradually coming to see, however, that as most other countries use Centigrade, and since it is much more convenient for most branches of science, it would really be better if we could change over and use it too. It is now used in British weather forecasts and is gradually being used more in other fields.

Here is the way to change Fahrenheit figures into Centigrade:
Subtract 32, multiply by 5, and divide by 9.
So 100° F into Centigrade would work out like this:

$$100 - 32 = 68 \times 5 = 340 \div 9 = 37 \cdot 7° \text{ C}$$
(38° to the nearest decimal point).

To change Centigrade into Fahrenheit you do it the other way round:

Multiply by 9, divide by 5 and add 32.
So 38° C becomes $38 \times 9 = 342 \div 5 = 68 \cdot 4 + 32 = 100 \cdot 4°$ F.

For your guidance:

97° F = 36·1° C	102° F = 38·8° C
98° F = 36·6° C	103° F = 39·4° C
99° F = 37·2° C	104° F = 40° C
100° F = 37·7° C	105° F = 40·5° C
101° F = 38·3° C	

Temperature

The temperature of a ward or sick room should be about 18° C (65° F) unless the doctor orders it to be higher, which may be so with children, old people, or people suffering from diseases of the lungs or chest.

A thermometer is an instrument used to record temperatures.

A clinical thermometer, used for taking the temperature of the body, consists of a narrow glass tube with a bulb containing mercury and a stem, up the centre of which is a tiny, hollow tube. Divisions or degrees from 95 to 110° F are marked on the stem by black lines so that the height of the mercury is easily seen. The space between each degree is divided into five smaller spaces, each representing two points. As the mercury in the tube becomes heated, it expands and rises up the tube, when it can be seen as a thin silver thread. A rectal thermometer has a special thick rounded bulb. There is also a universal type which can be used for any method, but if used rectally must be very clearly marked and kept for this purpose only.

The normal temperature of the body is 36 to 37° C (97 to 99° F), and varies very little in health.

Unless a patient is very ill, when his temperature is recorded four hourly or oftener, it is taken morning and evening, though this practice is often discarded after the temperature has been normal for some days, unless the patient develops fresh symptoms.

The temperature of the body may be taken in the mouth, in the axilla or groin, or in the rectum. A nurse must always insert and remove a thermometer herself. She must thoroughly wash and disinfect it after use and hold it in position in the case of children, restless patients, and those who are unconscious or delirious.

Articles needed on a thermometer tray

Jar containing a thermometer
Bowl of cold water free from disinfectant, for rinsing the thermometer
Swabs for drying the thermometer

Receiver for used swabs
The temperature is recorded as a graph on a special chart ruled
for the purpose. This must be kept very accurately and neatly.

HOW TO TAKE THE TEMPERATURE

1. *In the mouth.* Do not give either a hot or a cold drink
immediately before taking the temperature by this method.

Wipe the thermometer. See that the mercury has been shaken
down to below 95° F. Place the bulb under the tongue and close
the lips, telling the patient to be careful not to bite it.

NEVER take the temperature in the mouth in the case of young
children or of patients who are delirious, unconscious or who
have difficult breathing.

2. *In the axilla, i.e. under the arm.* Wipe the axilla with a swab.
Place the thermometer in position and see that it is not in contact
with any clothing or with a hot bottle. Draw the patient's arm
across the chest. Leave for at least 3 minutes.

This method should not be used immediately after the patient
has had a hot bath.

3. *In the rectum.* This method is useful in the case of infants,
and after accidents in the case of adults, when it is not possible
to use any other method. It must not be used immediately after
an enema has been given. A rectal thermometer should always
be kept in a specially marked container and should be greased
before it is inserted.

The temperature in the rectum is half a degree higher than in
the mouth, and in the mouth it is half a degree higher than in the
axilla or groin.

All thermometers should be left in position for at least twice as
long as the time stated on them. The interval is used for counting
the pulse and respirations.

In cases where an unexpected temperature occurs, the nurse
should retake it with another thermometer.

Immediately after use, hold the thermometer firmly between
the thumb and first finger of the right hand and flick from the
wrist to shake the mercury down. Then wash it in cold water,

wipe it and place it bulb downwards in a jar containing a suitable disinfectant. The bulb should be protected by a swab of cotton wool placed in the bottom of the jar. Each patient should have a separate thermometer. Sometimes it is thought better to store thermometers dry, in which case they will be cleaned in an antiseptic, dried, and put away in a container.

Terms used in connection with an abnormal temperature

A subnormal temperature is one below 36° C (96·8° F). This occurs when the blood pressure is very low, as in shock or after severe bleeding, or near death; when a person has been subjected to severe cold over a long period, especially if this is accompanied by malnutrition; and when a patient's temperature is deliberately reduced to 30° C, or even lower, during operations (hypothermia).

Pyrexia is what is usually meant by fever—a temperature over 37·2° C (99° F) rising to about 40° C (104° F).

Hyperpyrexia, higher still, is very rare except in malaria, or occasionally before death from some brain disease.

RIGOR

A rigor is an acute attack of shivering which may occur at the onset, or during the course, of an acute infection like pneumonia or meningitis. It has three stages.

Cold stage, in which the patient is blue, cold and shivering.

Hot stage, in which the patient is flushed, with dry skin, severe headache, full bounding pulse and rising temperature.

Sweating stage, in which there is profuse perspiration, the temperature falls rapidly and usually the pulse and general condition improve.

A rigor is always very serious and must be reported at once.

Shivering without a rise of temperature or sweating may be due to cold, fatigue or emotion.

Treatment of a rigor

When a rigor commences the nurse should place a warm

blanket next to the patient and a hot water bottle at his feet. More blankets may be piled on the bed until the shivering stops. The temperature should be taken in the axilla.

When the hot stage is reached the blankets should be removed and a cold drink be given. A cold compress may be placed on the forehead. During this stage the temperature is recorded every fifteen minutes. If it rises above 40·5° C (105° F) tepid sponging may be ordered.

Take the temperature again to note the limit which the pyrexia has reached.

When the patient begins to sweat sponge him down with warm water taking care not to chill him and change his clothing as often as may be necessary. The rigor may well exhaust the patient and his colour and pulse must be carefully watched. If a stimulant has been ordered it may be given at the end of the rigor and if the patient is then made comfortable he may sleep. During the course of a rigor the patient is never left alone.

The temperatures should be charted in red ink and the word 'Rigor' added.

SPONGING

Sponging is a measure which may be undertaken to reduce the temperature of the body in fever by $1\frac{1}{2}°$ to 2° F, and for its soothing effect on the patient.

Sponging has a cooling effect because it increases the amount of evaporation of moisture from the surface of the body, therefore the skin should be left damp.

Articles required for tepid sponging :

Clean, warm clothing
The patient's own bath blankets
Clinical thermometer
Large washing bowl
Water at 32° C (90° F), which may be allowed to cool to
24° C (75° F)

84

Bath thermometer
Two jugs, one of hot and one of cold water
Pail for change of water
Five sponges
Bowl to receive surplus water from sponge
Small bowl of iced water with compress for forehead
Ice cubes in bowl
The patient's brush and comb

Method

Place screens round the bed and close the windows to ensure privacy and prevent draughts.

Gently roll one bath blanket under the patient and cover him with the other.

Soak, squeeze lightly, and place a cold sponge in each axilla and on each groin.

Sponge and dry the face and, if the temperature is very high, place a cold compress on the forehead.

Using the sponges alternately and with long sweeping strokes sponge the arms in turn, then the body and legs.

Do not dry the skin, but leave it damp in order to allow cooling of the surface.

Take the temperature and compare it with that taken before the sponging. Stop treatment when it has fallen 2 degrees.

Wait until the skin is dry.

Remove the bottom blanket, straightening the bottom sheet and drawsheet.

Put a clean nightgown on the patient.

Brush and comb the hair with as little disturbance as possible.

Remove the upper bath blanket and cover with a sheet and blanket.

Give a suitable drink, e.g. lemonade, and take the temperature again, half an hour later.

The procedure should take about twenty minutes, and during this time the patient should be moved as little as possible.

The Pulse

A good indication of a patient's condition is the wave of movement which passes along the wall of an artery every time the heart beats. It is felt wherever an artery passes over a bone fairly near the skin. The radial artery is the best example of this.

Counting the pulse

Lay the arm on the bed with the elbow and wrist slightly flexed and place three fingers on the hollow so formed over the artery.

Do not count the pulse immediately after exertion and, in the case of nervous patients, keep on counting for a longer period than the usual time of one minute.

A nurse must notice the frequency, quality and regularity of the pulse.

By *frequency* is meant the number of beats in a given time. This should be about 120 per minute in the case of a small child; 72 per minute in the case of an adult; 60 per minute in the case of an old person.

By *quality* is meant the strength of the pulse, e.g. full and bounding in some forms of heart disease, thin and thready in collapse and haemorrhage.

A pulse is said to be:

Regular when the beats are equal in strength and when the pause between them is always of the same length.

Irregular when the beats vary in force and rhythm. This occurs in some forms of serious heart disease.

Intermittent when there is an occasional dropped beat.

Running when the beats are so rapid that they cannot be counted; this may occur after prolonged bleeding.

A nurse must always report any abnormal pulse to the sister or nurse in charge of the ward *especially* when she is keeping a quarter hourly pulse chart after accident or operation. A rising pulse rate may be the only indication of internal haemorrhage, and the nurse taking it may be the only one to know until it is too late. She must report it at once if the pulse rate is higher than the last time she took it. As a general rule, the weaker the pulse, the more dangerous the condition of the patient, while a falling temperature with an increase in the pulse rate is a very serious sign.

The Respiration

The normal respiration rate is between 16 and 20 breaths a minute.

They should be counted when the patient is unaware that this is being done, by keeping the fingers on the wrist as though still counting the pulse.

A nurse should notice whether they are quick, noisy or quiet, shallow or deep, difficult or easy, regular or irregular.

Breathing should be quiet and deep, but in some diseases it alters to rest the affected part.

It is *shallow* in cases of shock, collapse, peritonitis and pleurisy.

It is *quicker* in children, in feverish conditions and as a result of emotion and exertion.

It is *slower* in brain disease and head injury.

It is *noisy* in chest disease and apoplexy.

The term *dyspnoea* is used in connection with difficult breathing.

Sighing is a sign that the body is not receiving a sufficient amount of oxygen and occurs in shock and collapse.

Cheyne-Stokes breathing is a peculiar form of breathing occurring in cycles. It is always a very grave sign and can often be heard shortly before death in diseases of the vital organs, e.g. the heart and brain.

A nurse must draw the attention of the sister or nurse in charge of the ward to any abnormal sounds heard in connection with a patient's breathing.

GIVING AND RECEIVING REPORTS

The object of giving and receiving reports is to ensure that information necessary for the proper treatment and well-being

87

of the patient is passed on to the person who is in charge of the ward for the time being. It is also essential that accurate records should be available for the hospital files.

Writing Ward Reports

In writing ward reports, a record should be made of:

1. The date.
2. The number of patients in the ward and the number of empty beds.
3. Particulars of any new patients admitted, their name, age and the time admitted.
4. Whether the new patients have been seen by a doctor, and the doctor's name.
5. Particulars of any patient who has died.
6. Particulars of any patient who has been discharged, or who is to have an operation or a special examination, with full instructions as to time and preparation.
7. Any treatments given or ordered, or to be discontinued, any alterations in diet.
8. Information as to whether dangerously ill patients have been visited and, if so, at what time.
9. An accurate account of any drugs given and their effect on the patient and the time the next dose is due.
10. The nature of any dressings carried out, e.g. removal of stitches, renewals of dressings, re-packing of wounds.
11. The nature of any patient's pain and the steps taken to relieve it.
12. The time and nature of any vomiting and its relationship to food.
13. The amount and character of any sleep.
14. The quantity and nature of any nourishment taken, especially fluids.
15. Bowel and bladder action and, when necessary, the amount of urine passed.
16. Whether specimens have been sent to the laboratory.

17. Information as to the temperature, pulse and respiration of any patient who is not convalescent.

Do not use abbreviations except those you *know* are accepted and allowed.

Sign the report with your full name.

The Duties of the Night Nurse

She receives the report from the sister in charge of the ward and *makes sure* that she understands the nature of her patients' illness and the treatment they will require.

She sees to it that her supplies of medicines, drugs, oxygen, dressings, food, linen and other stores are ample for the night.

She then goes to the bedsides of the patients, attending to their comfort and their needs, adjusting pillows and bandages, renewing dressings, giving drinks, carrying out the treatments which have been ordered and taking the four-hourly temperatures.

Although a patient may need drugs to relieve his pain, or to help him to sleep, there is much that you, the night nurse, can do for him.

See that the ward is as quiet as possible. Wear shoes that make no sound. Get to know the loose floorboard, the squeaky trolley, the window that rattles in a high wind, and be prepared for it. Sound carries at night so be careful in the sluice and the kitchen.

There should be enough light for you to see your way about the ward, but no light should shine directly into a patient's face. Learn to use your torch so that only indirect light falls on the patient.

The ward should be warm, but not stuffy, and there should be no draughts.

If, after this, a patient is still wakeful, consider the following possible causes:

Unfamiliar surroundings	Feeling hungry or thirsty
Uncomfortable bed	Hearing others snoring
Feeling too hot	Difficulty in breathing
Feeling too cold	Pain
Wanting to pass water	Feeling worried or anxious

Offer the patient a bedpan or a urinal. Pull the drawsheet through so that he has a cool piece to lie on. Brush out any crumbs and see that the bottom sheet is free of creases. Shake up his pillows and loosen the clothes over his feet and chest. If he is allowed to have them bring him a hot water bottle and a hot milk drink. Often changing a patient's position and massaging his pressure areas will help him to relax sufficiently to fall asleep.

If he has pain, or difficulty in breathing, make him as comfortable as you can and let night sister know.

Perhaps he is worried about his family at home, or anxious about some treatment he is to have. Try to get him to tell you about it. The telling will ease his mind, and you may be able to reassure him. In any case, make a careful report about it to night sister on her next round, and to day sister in the morning, so that everything possible may be done to remove the worry.

When night sister comes round report to her any patients who are still not sleeping, or whose pulse is weakening, or who have a raised temperature, or any disturbing symptom such as a troublesome cough. For patients who are likely to receive drugs put their charts ready, and prepare a hypodermic tray. The drugs should be readily available, but kept locked up until night sister arrives.

The night nurse helps with the ward work as arranged with the ward sister, attends to the patients' needs throughout the night and then, in the early morning, helps with washings and bed-making, and in some cases with breakfast.

She sees to the tidying and ventilation of the ward and annexes, writes her account of the night's happenings, and gives a verbal report to the sister when she comes to take charge of the ward in the morning.

The Routine Care of the Patient

As she performs each of her duties carefully and quietly the nurse will learn to observe the patient so well that she will be able to report the slightest change, knowing that even those symptoms which appear to her most trivial may throw light on the patient's condition and help the doctor in his diagnosis and prescription of treatment.

A nurse should record:

1. The patient's temperature, pulse and respiration, noting carefully any changes, e.g. a raised temperature with a quick, feeble pulse.
2. The quantity and nature of any nourishment taken.
3. The amount and character of any sleep obtained.
4. The amount of fluid taken in and the output in urine and vomit.

SIGNS OF ILLNESS

Malaise :   A general feeling of not being well, such as head-ache, aching of the back and limbs, shivering, loss of appetite.

Posture :   The position in which the patient lies in bed, e.g. the patient may lie on the side of the pain so that pressure may give relief, or in the case of abdominal pain he may draw his knees up to avoid pressure on the painful part, or he may be afraid to move.

Appearance :   The face usually shows signs of pain.

It may be *expressionless* when the patient is unconscious, or it may be *pinched and drawn* and the eyes may be sunken in their sockets when fluid has been lost to the body through haemorrhage, vomiting and excessive perspiration. The patient may look anxious and frightened.

Skin changes :   In fever the skin is hot and dry, then later moist, with a falling temperature.

Rashes :   These may indicate the onset of an infectious disease, or increased sensitiveness to some food or drug.

Colour :   Cyanosis or blueness of the lips, ears, tips of the nails, etc., may be due to a lack of oxygen in the tissues associated with disease of the heart or lungs.

Pallor : This may be due to disease, e.g. anaemia, nephritis, or to shock and faintness.

Flushing : This may be due to raised temperature, but is normal after an anaesthetic.

Jaundice : This shows as a yellow discoloration of the skin and conjunctiva. It is usually a symptom of gall stones or liver disease.

The tongue : A furred tongue may be a sign of digestive disorder or of infection.

Vomiting : A nurse should notice the nature of any material vomited, the time when it occurs, and the quantity (p. 117).

Vomiting and diarrhoea together produce *dehydration*, a word which means the loss of water from the body. This can happen very quickly, especially in young children, and is always serious.

Cough : If it is hard, dry and painful, it may be due to pneumonia. If it is brassy and wheezing it may be due to a serious condition, aneurysm of the aorta. If it is hacking it may be due to obstruction of the air passages.

Frothy blood which appears after coughing is from the lungs.

Sputum : The quantity and type of sputum should be noted (p. 117), i.e. the presence of blood or pus, clear or foul smelling.

The abdomen : Distension of the abdomen apart, of course, from pregnancy, may be due to tumours, gas or a distended bladder which may need catheterizing.

Swelling : This may accompany inflammation following injury or infection, or it may be due to accumulation of fluid in the tissues in heart or kidney disease.

Cries: Unusual cries may accompany brain disease, diseases of the joints, and 'bad dreams'.

Any abnormalities of the *urine* and *faeces* must be reported; also discharges from the *eyes*, *ears* and *nose*.

If the patient is having any special treatment the nurse should watch for and report any reactions, e.g. headache, vomiting, etc.

11

Giving Medicines and Drugs

The enrolled nurse may occasionally be asked to check a drug for a trained nurse, but she is not as a rule asked to give Dangerous Drugs. These are kept in a special, locked cupboard and only the sister or trained staff nurse in charge of the ward keeps the key.

They can be given to the patient only when ordered by a doctor on a written and signed prescription and their administration must be checked by a second person.

A careful record, which must be kept for at least two years, must give the name of the patient, the amount of the drug given, the date and time when given and the name of the witness as well as of the nurse who has given the drug.

Medicines

These must always be kept in their own cupboard, apart from lotions used externally. They may be given:
1. By mouth
2. By rectum
3. By injection
4. By inunction, i.e. rubbing into the skin
5. By inhalation

Before giving medicines, the pupil nurse should study a few of the abbreviations commonly used in prescriptions.

94

Giving Medicines and Drugs

Abbreviation	Latin Term	English Term
a.c.	ante cibum	before food
p.c.	post cibum	after food
m.	mane	morning
n.	nocte	in the night
b.d.	bis die	twice a day
t.d.s.	ter die sumendus	three times a day
t.i.d.	ter in die	three times a day
q.h.	quartis horis	four hourly
stat.	statim	immediately
s.o.s.	si opus sit	if necessary and once only
p.r.n.	pro re nata	whenever necessary
ad lib.	ad libitum	freely, at pleasure
ex aq.	ex aqua	in water
c.	cum	with
p.r.	per rectum	by the rectum
rep.	repetatur	to be repeated
s.s.	semis	half
Cat.	Cataplasma	Poultice
Gutt.	Gutta	Drop
Mist.	Mistura	Mixture
Ol.	Oleum	Oil
Pil.	Pilula	Pill
Pulv.	Pulvis	Powder
Ung.	Unguentum	Ointment

When measuring medicines it is necessary to remember that according to the *liquid measure* there are:

> 60 minims in a drachm
> 8 drachms in a fluid ounce
> 20 fluid ounces in a pint
> 17 minims in 1 millilitre or ml.; a millilitre is almost exactly a cubic centimetre (c.c.)
> 1,000 millilitres, or 1 litre, in 35 fluid ounces

According to the *dry measure* there are:

> 60 grains in 1 drachm
> 8 drachms in 1 ounce
> 15 grains in 1 gramme
> 1,000 grammes, or 1 kilogram, in 2·2 pounds

Medicines and aperients are given only when ordered by a doctor, and a nurse should never give any dose unless she is sure it is the correct one. If she is in any doubt, she must consult the doctor or, if she is in hospital, the ward sister or charge nurse, and verify her instructions.

The correct medicine is given at the *exact* time ordered and the nurse must watch for and report any after effects, e.g. headache, vomiting, slow pulse, etc.

Remember this rule: 'The right medicine and the right dose to the right patient at the right time.'

As a rule medicines are given about twenty minutes after a meal.

Aperients acting slowly, e.g. vegetable laxatives, should be given *last thing at night*, and those acting quickly, e.g. salts, which should be given with a cup of tea, *first thing* in the morning.

Articles needed on a medicine tray

Medicines as ordered
Patients' prescription cards
Well-marked glass measures, ounce and minim
Well-marked china oil cups
Spoon
Glass jug of cold water
Glass bowl of warm water
Glass cloth
Rod for stirring medicines with a sediment
A bowl of water for washing the glasses
A clean cloth for drying them
Orange juice
Sweets
Straws

TO POUR OUT A MEDICINE

1. Check that the medicine in the bottle corresponds to that on the patient's prescription card. Check that you are administering it to the right patient. If a patient is new, or you are new to the ward, ask the patient his name before you give the medicine.

2. Place the finger over the cork and shake the medicine by inverting the bottle a few times. This prevents the heavier ingredients from settling at the bottom.

3. With the little finger of the left hand, remove the cork and hold it, as shown in Fig. 10. Do not put it down, as it would come into contact with dust and germs, or might get lost. Hold the medicine glass between the thumb and finger of the left hand.

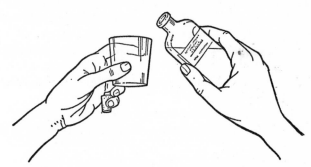

FIG. 10. THE CORRECT WAY TO POUR MEDICINE

4. Holding the bottle in the right hand with the label uppermost and the glass at eye level, measure to the lowest point of the curve which appears on the surface of the liquid, level with the marking on the measure. *Always* pour from the back of the bottle, *never* over the label, lest it becomes discoloured and illegible.

5. Carry the medicine to the bedside on a tray, and see that the patient takes it at once. Never leave it with the patient. A medicine, once poured out, is never returned to the bottle, but is thrown away. Any re-labelling of bottles is done by the dispenser.

6. If a medicine has an unpleasant taste, a sweet or a drink of orange juice in cold water usually can be given after it.

7. Medicine must *never* be used from an unlabelled bottle. If the nurse is unsure about the substance in a bottle it must be sent back to the dispensary. Any bottles that are nearly

empty should be put into the dispensary basket and not be allowed to run out.

8. Bottles should be wiped and put away in their correct places.

Any oil can be made pleasanter by pouring into the glass a little orange or lemon juice, then the oil, then some more fruit juice. Tell the patient to swallow it quickly. A biscuit or piece of dry toast to follow will remove any oil left in the mouth.

Pills, capsules or tablets can, as a rule, be swallowed whole with a drink of water, or pills can be crushed and given in jam.

Powders and cachets may be placed on the tongue and washed down with a drink of water.

Effervescing powders should be given in water and swallowed when effervescing.

Medicines containing iron should be offered with a straw, or they will stain the teeth.

There are hundreds of medicines and drugs in use today, but they all come under one group or another according to their use.

The main groups are:

1. *Anaesthetics.* These act on the nervous system and produce either loss of consciousness (if general) or loss of sensation (if local), e.g. ether and its variations; cocaine and similar drugs.

2. *Analgesics* and *antipyretics* often work together to relieve pain and lower high temperatures. They are given in rheumatic conditions and for mild aches and pains, e.g. aspirin; codeine; Butazolidine.

3. *Antibiotics* form perhaps the biggest group of all now, and more are added constantly. They stop the growth of bacteria in the body, each drug being effective against one particular type of germ. The best known are the various types of *penicillin* and *streptomycin*.

N.B.—A rash due to sensitivity to some of these drugs may occur in nurses who have to handle them often, so care must be taken to see that the needle is firmly attached to the syringe when giving an injection; rubber gloves should be worn, and a mask to protect the face. Hands and arms should be washed as soon as the procedure is finished.

4. *Antihistamine* drugs help people with allergic conditions like asthma or hay fever or irritating skin conditions like nettle rash, e.g. Benadryl; Ancolan.

5. *Aperients* produce bowel action, e.g. cascara, Dulcolax.

6. *Diuretics* increase the output of urine by stimulating the kidneys, e.g. mersalyl, Lasix.

7. *Expectorants* are mixtures that make coughing easier and so enable the patient to bring up the irritating sputum.

8. *Hypnotics* make people feel sleepy. They include barbiturates like Luminal and Medinal, and all the tablets that are given at night to patients who need something to help them rest properly.

Narcotics are stronger than hypnotics. They kill severe pain, relieve fear and anxiety, and so enable the patient to sleep. They include many of the Dangerous Drugs, such as morphine, opium and pethidine.

Injections

Hypodermic injections are given into the subcutaneous tissue and drugs given by this route act quickly. Many drugs given by this method are controlled by the Dangerous Drugs Act; therefore it is the usual rule in most hospitals that all hypodermic injections are checked by a second person and that the drug, the dose given, and the date and time of the administration are recorded.

Articles needed on a hypodermic tray :

A 1 or 2 ml. capacity syringe
Hypodermic needles, sizes 17 or 20
These generally come from a Central Sterile Supply Department, ready to use
A piece of sterile gauze on which to rest the syringe and needle
A swab moistened with spirit or cetrimide for cleaning the skin
A receiver
The patient's prescription card
Before giving a hypodermic injection, the hands must be washed and dried.

If the syringe has been stored in spirit it must be rinsed in sterile water before being used.

Place the syringe in the receiver with the needle resting on a swab which has been dipped in spirit.

If the drug is to be taken from a rubber-capped bottle, the rubber cap must be cleaned with spirit, the needle inserted, and a little air injected before drawing up the drug. Turn the bottle upside down while you draw out the exact amount of the drug.

If the drug is in a glass ampoule, wash the glass first with spirit, then hold it with the swab and use a file to cut the neck.

Tell the patient what you are going to do, and what effect the drug should have, e.g. make him sleepy, or make his pain easier.

Cleanse the skin with spirit and take up a fleshy fold of skin free from veins, usually on the arm or on the thigh.

Holding this firmly between the thumb and finger of the left hand, insert the needle quickly and gently in a slightly upward direction, and give the drug by pressing the piston home.

With a swab over the puncture, withdraw the needle quickly and massage the skin to promote absorption of the drug.

The secret of giving painless injections lies in having a perfectly sharp needle and inserting it *quickly*.

THE ADMINISTRATION OF INSULIN

Insulin is supplied in rubber-capped bottles in strengths of 20, 40 and 80 units. It is particularly important that insulin is stored in a cool place, and that the syringe and needle are stored in alcohol or kept dry.

Before use the syringe is rinsed in sterile water and the rubber cap wiped over with spirit and pierced by a needle.

In most syringes, the ml. is divided into 20 subdivisions, there-fore each subdivision will contain:

1 unit if the label on the bottle is 20 units per ml.
2 units if it is 40 units per ml. and
4 units if it is 80 units per ml.

There are many types of insulin; some have a quick effect and some an effect spread over 24 hours. The dose and type must be carefully checked for each separate patient.

The site of the injection should be changed frequently and a second injection should not be given in the same place within 48 hours.

Insulin should be given half an hour before the meal specified, which usually is breakfast and tea. Soluble insulin begins to act on the blood sugar within 30 minutes of being injected and its action ceases after 6 to 10 hours.

Globin insulin with zinc begins to act in 2 hours and its action continues for 18 to 24 hours.

Protamine zinc insulin does not begin to act for 10 hours, and it continues to act for 24 to 36 hours.

In these cases daily injections only are necessary; but the doctor will always give exact instructions.

Insulin can also be given by mouth, in tablet form, e.g. Rastinon.

INTRAMUSCULAR INJECTIONS

When a large amount of a drug has to be given, or if it contains something likely to irritate the nerve endings under the skin, it will be given deep down into a muscle. These points must be remembered:

1. Since the drug has to be given some way from the surfaces, a longer, stronger needle must be used than for hypodermic injections, attached to a syringe large enough to contain the full dose, usually 10 or 20 ml.

2. There is grave danger of the needle damaging a nerve— usually the sciatic nerve—or even the periosteum of a bone, or of entering a blood vessel, if the site is not carefully chosen. If the buttock is chosen, an imaginary cross is drawn over it and the injection given into the upper, outer angle. Some doctors, however, prefer that this region should not be used at all, and like the injection to be given into the side of the thigh, where there are no important vessels or nerves. It may be given into the front of the

thigh, or into the deltoid on the shoulder if the patient is well covered. It is best to ask the ward sister to look at the patient and do as she advises.

3. Everything used must be sterile.
4. The nurse must wash her hands thoroughly before giving the injection.

If glass syringes are sterilized on the ward, clean thoroughly first in cold and then in warm soapy water, running it several times through the needle to clean it; then take to pieces, wrap the glass barrel in gauze, and lay the parts in cold water. Bring to the boil and boil for 3 minutes.

Disposable syringes, now commonly used, are of course thrown away after use.

Drugs Given by Inhalation

Inhalations are useful in cases of sore throat, laryngitis, irritating cough and nasal congestion.

Moist inhalations

These are given by means of a Nelson's inhaler.

Required, tray containing:

Nelson's inhaler
Jug of hot water
Friars' balsam or menthol crystals
Minim measure or teaspoon
Piece of gauze to protect the glass mouthpiece
Flannel cover
Bowl

Method. Heat the inhaler with hot water and then pour this away. Fill with water just off the boil to a slightly lower level than that of the airway, which must be turned away from the patient. Add to this the drug ordered, usually one drachm of friars' balsam (tincture of benzoin) or two menthol crystals.

Immediately clean with spirit the spoon or measure that has been used.

Put the inhaler in a flannel bag, stand it on a tray in a bowl and place in on a bed table. Prop the patient up and arrange the inhaler in front of him. Make sure that the airway is turned *away* from him, otherwise if he tilts the inhaler he may scald himself. Wrap a piece of gauze round the mouthpiece of the inhaler to protect the patient's mouth from the hot glass. Put a shawl or light blanket round his shoulders. Tell him to breathe in through his mouth and out through his nose.

If no Nelson's inhaler is available, make a funnel with a folded towel round the mouthpiece of a straight jug, to prevent the steam from escaping.

Provide a sputum mug, as the inhalation may make the patient cough.

Never leave a child or a restless patient alone with a hot inhaler.

STEAM TENTS

A steam tent is used when it is necessary to maintain a warm, moist atmosphere round the patient. The temperature in the tent should be from 18 to 24° C (65 to 75° F) or as ordered.

It is made by placing a large screen round the head of the bed and covering over the top with a sheet which must be fastened to the screen covers. Sufficient space must be left inside the tent for the nurse to attend to the patient.

Steam enters the tent by means of an electric kettle with a long spout.

This may stand on a low stool. The position of the kettle does not matter so long as:

(*a*) It is out of reach of the patient so that he cannot touch any part of it; or be scalded by it.

(*b*) It is placed so that sufficient steam enters the area where the patient is breathing so that he inhales the now warmed, damp air.

(*c*) It does not interfere with other nursing duties or stand where anyone can fall over it.

ALWAYS ASK THE WARD SISTER WHERE SHE WANTS IT PLACED.

There should be a metal gutter along the lower border of the spout to direct the condensed water from the steam into a small bucket which hangs under the spout.

The kettle must not be allowed to boil dry, and boiling water should be used for re-filling.

A thermometer should hang inside the tent at the level of the patient's head to record the temperature of the air he is breathing. This should not exceed 24° C (75° F).

Oxygen Administration

Oxygen, supplied in cylinders, is a heart and respiratory stimulant which is given to relieve breathlessness and cyanosis in cases where the patient cannot take in enough oxygen from the air by ordinary breathing, as for example, in severe shock. Perhaps parts of the lungs are blocked, as in pneumonia, or the heart is not strong enough to pump the blood round the whole circulation. A lot of red blood cells may have been lost, as after haemorrhage, or may not be working properly, as in shock or anaemia.

The gas may be turned on by means of a handle with a fine adjustment valve. By means of this the rate of flow of the oxygen from the cylinder may be controlled.

From the cylinder it passes through a rubber tube with a glass connection, to a face mask or two rubber catheters which are inserted into the patient's nostrils.

Oxygen dries the respiratory passages, so, in order to avoid irritating the mucous membranes, it should be moistened by being passed through water in a Woulfe's bottle. This has two bent glass tubes passing through two corks in the neck. *The longer tube* is connected by rubber tubing to the oxygen cylinder, and *the shorter tube* by tubing and a glass connection to the face mask or to the two nasal catheters. The end of this tube must always be above the level of the water so that oxygen and not water enters the nose. Test it before attaching it to the patient.

Disposable masks

Transparent plastic face masks are now more frequently used for giving oxygen than any other form of apparatus. A commonly used type is the Polymask which consists of a double bag of transparent polythene with a flexible wire frame that can be fitted to the patient's face. It is kept in position by thin cords which hitch the bag to the patient's ears. Oxygen passes from the cylinder between the layers of the bag and reaches the patient through two small holes in the inner layer; there are also ventilation holes in the outer layer. The mask is destroyed after use.

The *B.L.B. mask* is a rubber mask which fits over the nose or the nose and mouth and is held in position by means of a strap round the head. The mask is connected to a breathing bag, and then by means of narrow tubing to the oxygen cylinder.

After use the *rubber mask and bag* can be sterilized by boiling in plain water for three minutes, and the *metal connection* by placing it in antiseptic, e.g. Dettol, then rinsing in water. The whole should be thoroughly dried before it is put away.

Nasal catheters

These are used when a face mask is unsuitable, as, for example, where there are facial injuries, and when an oxygen tent is not available.

Clean the patient's nose with moist swabs. Lubricate the ends of the catheters with petroleum jelly or if need be with cocaine ointment, and pass them for about 2 inches along the floor of the nose.

They are kept in position by narrow pieces of strapping. Another method is to use a Tudor Edwards spectacle frame. The catheters should be changed whenever they become blocked with mucus.

Oxygen should flow from the cylinder at the rate of about four litres a minute and the exact volume of oxygen being plied is measured by a flowmeter or, in its absence, by the bubbles on the surface of the water. These should be so rapid that they can only just be counted. In some cases, a flowmeter is combined with the humidifier.

A new oxygen cylinder should be opened outside the ward. No grease or lubricant should be applied to any part lest an explosion occurs, neither should the cylinder be allowed to fall on the floor.

The tubing must not be allowed to kink and the nurse must see that the oxygen is flowing from the cylinder at the right rate before she brings the cylinder to the bedside.

All empty cylinders should be marked at once and replaced with full ones.

Oxygen tent

This apparatus is made of transparent plastic, and in several different sizes to fit over cradle, cot, or bed. The use of the tent allows for a continuous high concentration of oxygen to be maintained. It is specially used for patients who are seriously ill. There are openings in the tent through which the nurse can put her arms when attending to the patient. These are closed with zip fasteners when not in use. The apparatus includes an extra large oxygen cylinder, and a refrigeration unit, which cools the air. The temperature of the tent should not be allowed to rise above 21° C (70° F).

NOTE. No naked flame may be allowed near an oxygen tent or cylinder as there is grave danger of fire and explosion. Not only the nursing staff should know this, but the patients also, since a patient smoking a cigarette may inadvertently walk near the tent if he is not informed. No toys which can emit sparks may be allowed in a children's ward when an oxygen tent is in use.

12

General Nursing Procedures

In many of the procedures you will have to learn to carry out, you will have to prepare and use hot lotions.

Never get careless about testing the temperature of these lotions.

Always use a proper lotion thermometer and never trust to luck or your own sensations when using anything which will go on to or into a patient's body. In most cases lotions are used at body temperature or a little above—not more than 38° C (100° F). If you are in doubt about what is meant by 'hot' in treatments that cannot very well be tested with a thermometer, such as hot kaolin poultices, then, and only then, test with the back of your hand or elbow. If it is too hot for you, it is too hot for your patient.

The highest temperature for a hot soak for, e.g. a septic finger, is 55° C (130° F). Above that, a scald can result.

For want of that extra moment of care, a scald can be inflicted which may cause untold suffering to an already sick person.

Bathing and Irrigation of the Eye

Bathing the eye is done to relieve the pain of styes, etc., and inflammation of the eyelids.

The *method* most commonly employed is to tie a piece of boracic lint round the bowl of a wooden spoon, dip it into a basin of hot water 49° C (120° F) and lift it towards the eye.

The patient sits in front of the bowl which is placed on a table or bed table and wears a plastic cape and towel round the neck. The treatment is carried out for about fifteen minutes and repeated as often as is necessary.

Irrigation of the eyes is carried out by means of an undine (a specially shaped flask).

Required:

Shoulder blanket
Plastic cape
Dressing towel
Jug of lotion at 38° C (100° F), e.g. saline 1 teaspoonful to 1 pint water or boracic 2%
Lotion thermometer
Bowl of lotion containing the undine
Bowl containing swabs and eye pads
Wool pad for cheek
Receiver for used swabs
Receiver for used lotion

Method. Observe the strictest aseptic precautions throughout the preparations for, and during, the treatment.

Stand behind the patient, who should sit upright, his head well back and turned slightly towards the affected side. Put the waterproof cape and towel round his shoulders.

Place a receiver in a suitable position to catch the fluid and ask the patient to hold it steady.

Wipe the lids free of discharge—swabbing towards the outer corner of the eye and using each swab once only.

Open the eye very gently, pressing on the bone above the eye and not on the eye itself.

Pour the lotion over the cheek first, to accustom the patient to the feeling, then into the inner corner of the eye. Instruct him to move the eye up and down.

After all the lotion has been used, dry the eye and cheek gently with sterile swabs (a separate one for each).

Do not allow the patient to go into the cold air with the eye uncovered.

Poultices

Poultices provide a useful method of applying continuous heat to a part.

A *kaolin poultice* retains its heat for several hours, but care must be taken in its application or serious burns may result.

Required:

Poultice board
Old linen with the edges cut away at the corners
Single layer of gauze
Spatula in jug of boiling water
Kaolin in saucepan of boiling water

Tray containing:

Pad of wool
Bandage and safety pins
Receiver for old poultice
Olive oil in bowl of warm water
Swabs
Two warmed plates

Method. Loosen the lid and heat the kaolin by boiling the tin in a saucepan of water for about 20 minutes. Stir well. Lay the linen on the board and spread the kaolin on it with a heated spatula.

Cover with a single layer of gauze, turn in the edges, and carry it between the warmed plates to the patient's bedside.

Test on the back of the hand and apply gently over the affected area, then cover with warm wool and bandage in position.

Before renewing the poultice, any dry kaolin should be removed from the skin with a swab dipped in warm olive oil.

After the treatment has finished, keep the part covered for a day or two.

STARCH POULTICE

This poultice is useful for removing crusts in skin diseases. It should be ¾ inch thick and should be left on for six to twelve hours.

Required:

    1½ tablespoonfuls powdered starch
    1 teaspoonful boracic powder
    ½ pint boiling water
    Cold water to mix the starch and boracic powder to a thick cream
    Poultice board
    Old linen
    Mixing bowl
    Jug
    Spatula and spoon
    Kettle of boiling water
    Warm olive oil and swabs (for removing old poultice)
    Receiver for used swabs and old poultice
    Layer of old linen for covering poultice
    Plastic covering
    Bandage and safety pins

Method. Mix the starch and the boracic powder to a thick cream with a little cold water.

Stir in boiling water quickly until the starch is cooked and becomes thick and clear. When the starch is almost cold, spread the jelly on a piece of old linen and cover with a layer of old linen. Cover, and bandage in position.

Renew as directed.

Other Local Applications

Liniments are oily solutions containing turpentine, methyl salicylate or menthol.

Warm by standing in hot water, and rub in with the hand after the part has been washed, continuing to rub until the part is fairly dry and the skin reddened. The gentle warmth is comforting for stiff joints and 'rheumatic' pains in muscles.

Strapping and Elastoplast should be warmed, and snipped at the edges to prevent creasing.

Strapping the chest may be employed as a form of splinting to give relief in some cases of pleurisy and to support a fractured clavicle or ribs.

Removing strapping and Elastoplast can be very painful for the patient because the hairs on the skin are torn out with the plaster. To lessen this always shave the skin before applying Elastoplast in any quantity.

When you remove Elastoplast take a swab dipped in ether, raise a small corner of the Elastoplast, press the swab hard against the uncovered skin and rip the plaster back for a few inches. Move the swab close up against the plaster again, and rip back another section.

The cold of the ether distracts the patient's attention for a moment, while pressing hard on the skin keeps it tight, and by ripping the plaster rather than gently pulling it off the patient will hardly feel anything. Marks left on the skin after the Elastoplast has been taken off are easily removed by rubbing with a swab dipped in ether.

Paints, such as gentian violet, are used to control infection. They are applied to the skin with a wool swab and the area is left uncovered.

Ointments are often rubbed into the skin, e.g. zinc and castor oil ointment applied to the pressure areas of an incontinent patient. Others may be applied by spreading them on strips of old linen.

Lotions may be used as wet dressings, e.g. lead lotion to reduce the swelling of a sprain. The dressing is soaked in the lotion and applied without a bandage if possible, so that evaporation takes place. See that the dressing is kept wet all the time.

Other lotions, such as calamine to relieve skin irritation, are best swabbed on to the skin and left open to the air.

13

Nursing Duties Concerned
With Excretions

Urine

Urine, the waste matter from the kidneys, consists of 96%
water and 4% solids, of which 2% is urea.

The normal colour of urine is a clear, light amber.

The specific gravity is 1,015 to 1,025.

The reaction is slightly acid.

It should smell characteristic but not offensive.

The average quantity passed daily is 40 to 50 ounces, passed in
quantities of 10 ounces at a time every 4 hours.

Urine is tested on the admission of the patient to hospital to
assist in diagnosis, before an operation and to note the progress
of a disease and the effects of certain drugs.

It should be measured and tested daily in the following diseases:

> Heart disease
> Kidney disease
> Diabetes mellitus

and whenever the quantity appears to be excessive or diminishing.

During pregnancy it should be tested weekly so that any strain
on the kidneys can be detected early enough to give the mother
extra care.

The following abnormalities may be present in urine:

Albumin in nephritis or heart disease; occasionally in pregnancy.

Blood, Mucus, Pus in kidney and bladder diseases.

Sugar, Acetone and *Ketones* in diabetes.

Vessels into which urine is passed must be scrupulously clean and free from soda or the reaction will be rendered alkaline.

A nurse should note the colour, odour and deposit. A brick red dust indicates the presence of urates, and one similar to cayenne pepper, of uric acid.

To take a twenty-four hour specimen of urine

Empty the bladder at 8 a.m. and throw the urine away.

Save and measure all the urine passed, including that at 8 o'clock the next morning. This is all saved in a large bottle and sent to the laboratory. It may be asked for when tuberculosis of the kidney is suspected.

SIMPLE URINE TESTS

1. Note the colour, odour and deposit.
2. Take the reaction with litmus paper.
   If red litmus paper turns blue, the reaction is alkaline; if blue litmus paper turns red, it is acid.
3. Take the specific gravity by means of the urinometer.

With the new range of diagnostic reagents for urine testing called Albustix, Clinitest, etc, the work of the nurse has been made much easier, and the results of the tests much more accurate.

Full directions will be found with the tablets, but here are two examples.

1. *Albustix for the detection of protein (albumin).* (1) Dip test end of strip in urine and remove at once. (2) Compare colour of dipped end with colour scale. POSITIVE = The colour changes to green or blue. NEGATIVE = No colour change. Test end stays yellow. After comparing the test with the colour scale, write down the result.
2. *Clinitest for the detection of sugar.* Place 5 drops of urine in test tube. Rinse dropper and add 10 drops of water. Drop in one Clinitest tablet and watch reaction. 15 seconds after

boiling stops, shake tube gently and compare with Clinitest colour scale. NEGATIVE=Solution in test tube is blue. POSITIVE = Any colour other than blue. For degree compare with colour scale.

ABNORMALITIES OF MICTURITION

Difficult micturition or *retention of urine* may be due to an unaccustomed position in bed. It may be overcome by making the patient familiar with a particular position before undergoing an operation, by giving warm drinks and, where allowed, applying hot fomentations over the lower abdomen. If possible, allow the patient to sit over the side of the bed, or on a commode.

Only after all natural methods have failed should a catheter be passed.

Increased frequency of micturition is when the act of passing urine takes place oftener than once in four hours. This may be due to irritation, disease, pressure or anxiety.

Suppression of urine occurs when the kidneys fail to manufacture urine or when the ureters are blocked.

Incontinence is the failure of the bladder to retain urine. It occurs where there is paralysis of the lower half of the body, or in old or bedridden people where there is great weakness.

Retention with incontinence is due to stretching of the muscle round the neck of the bladder as a result of the bladder becoming over full. Urine dribbles away, yet some always remains in the bladder.

Enuresis or bed wetting is the incontinence of childhood. It may be due to faulty training, to nervous trouble, or to the child being cold in bed. See that he is well wrapped up and comfortable. Never scold him, but praise him when he has successfully spent a night dry.

Intake and output charts are kept for many patients suffering from kidney or heart diseases. The object of these is to record how well the patient's excretory organs are dealing with the amount of fluid he is taking. An accurate record conscientiously kept by the nursing staff is of great value to the doctor.

All the drinks given to the patient should be measured, and of course everything left. If a blood or saline transfusion is being given, the number of flasks must be noted. All urine or vomit is carefully measured and charted, and bowel motions or sweating noted.

CATHETERIZATION

Catheterization, the act of withdrawing urine from the bladder by means of a catheter, may be ordered by a doctor:

(*a*) Before an operation on the pelvic organs.

(*b*) In cases where the patient cannot pass urine naturally, e.g. after an operation or in cases of paralysis.

(*c*) When a specimen of urine is required for bacteriological examination.

As the bladder and its passages are very easily contaminated by germs catheterization should never be carried out unless it is absolutely necessary, and the most scrupulous aseptic precautions must be observed.

The articles needed are :

A bell lamp, where necessary, to provide a good light
Plastic square
Sterile towels
Sterile receiver for the urine
Sterile swabs
Sterile lotion for swabbing
Sterile catheters (at least two)
Sterile dissecting forceps
Receiver for used swabs ⎫
Receiver for used catheters ⎬ or disposal bags
Receiver for used forceps ⎭

Method. This is a sterile procedure.

Place the patient in the recumbent position with the knees flexed.

Turn back the bedclothes and cover the patient's shoulders and chest with a small blanket.

Place the plastic square under the patient's thighs.

Arrange the lamp to shine directly on to the vulva.

Wash your hands thoroughly and dry them on a clean towel. From now on your hands will become contaminated if they touch anything which is not sterile.

Turn back the bedclothes with your elbows.

Place the sterile towels over the patient's thighs and the sterile receiver between her legs.

With your left hand separate the labia. This hand continues to hold the labia apart throughout the procedure. It is now contaminated and on no account should you touch any of the sterile equipment with your left hand.

With your right hand swab the vulva in a downwards direction, using each swab once only. Start from the outer aspect and finish by swabbing the area around the urethra.

Pick up the catheter with the forceps in your right hand. Rest the end of the catheter in the sterile receiver.

Insert the tip gently into the urethra.

If it touches any part of the vulva before entering the urethra it becomes unsterile. Discard it immediately and take the second catheter.

Pass the catheter in for about two inches, until urine starts to flow into the receiver.

When the urine stops withdraw the catheter slowly.

Remove the receiver.

Dry the vulva with sterile swabs.

You may now use your left hand.

Remake the bed and leave the patient comfortable.

If a specimen is required for laboratory testing it should be collected in a sterile, screw-topped specimen bottle.

If a male patient is to be catheterized it will be done by a doctor or a male nurse. In addition to the above equipment they will need a sterile lubricant, such as sterile liquid paraffin. If the catheter is to be left in position after the procedure they will also need a spigot to close the end of the catheter, adhesive strapping and scissors.

Most hospitals now use disposable catheters which are supplied already sterilized in sealed plastic bags, and are thrown away after use.

Sputum

Sputum may be highly infectious and must be received into a disposable carton with a lid. Cartons should be burnt every day.

The nurse should note the amount of sputum expectorated, the colour, the appearance and the presence and nature of any abnormalities.

Vomit

The nurse should always save a specimen of vomited matter so that the following points about it may be noted: colour, quantity, consistency, frequency.

She should notice whether vomiting is preceded by nausea and retching, the time it occurs, whether it bears any relation to any meal or article of diet, if it is accompanied by pain or relieved by it, and whether it is projectile in character.

Bright yellow or greenish vomit which contains bile is a sign of liver disorder.

Greenish vomit often occurs after an anaesthetic.

Vomited blood may be blood which has been swallowed after tooth extraction, etc., or it may accompany disease of the stomach, duodenum or liver.

Faeces

Normally a stool occurs:	once a day
Quantity passed:	4 ounces
Consistency:	soft and solid
Odour:	inoffensive
Shape:	cylindrical
Colour:	light brown

Constipation, when a stool is passed less frequently than once in 48 hours, may be due to faulty habits, unsuitable diet or disease.

Diarrhoea, the too frequent emptying of the contents of the bowel, may be due to unsuitable food or to disease.

N.B.—All cases of abnormal stools must be reported to the sister or trained nurse in charge of the ward, and in private nursing to the doctor.

THE COLLECTION OF SPECIMENS

Faeces should be covered with a sheet of glass or a cloth wrung out in a disinfectant. Place the bedpan in the sluice in a specially ventilated cupboard or near the window.

Urine should be placed in a clean specimen glass and covered.

Sputum for examination must be expectorated into a special flask. No disinfectant should be added as this would interfere with the bacteriological findings.

Laboratory specimens should be sent away immediately they are obtained. They should be put in the special sterile container provided, using the special spatula provided to obtain a specimen (of faeces). They should be carefully labelled with the patient's name, the date and time obtained, and sent together with the pathological form.

The container must be very carefully sealed and packed and labelled 'Laboratory specimen'.

The nurse must wash her hands thoroughly after handling any excreta.

ENEMAS

An enema is a fluid preparation for injection into the rectum. It is given for the following reasons:
1. To empty the bowel of faeces.
2. To relieve distension.
3. To introduce drugs or extra fluids into the body.
4. To aid in diagnosis.

The type of enema which the enrolled nurse will most likely be required to give is the *simple enema* for the relief of constipation or to empty the bowel before an operation.

A nurse does not give an enema unless it has been ordered by the doctor.

Most hospitals now have disposable enemas. These are used according to the directions, which are simple. Disposable enemas only take a few minutes to give and therefore save a great deal of nurses' time. A few hospitals may still be using the old method.

Giving a simple enema (old method)

Plain water may be used, or a solution of soap and water made up from a stock solution kept in the ward.

Prepare a tray containing :

Plastic square and towel
Petroleum jelly
Gallipot containing a few swabs or pieces of old linen
Receiver for used swabs
Jug, containing the enema solution prepared to be given at
    38° C (100° F), standing in a bowl of hot water, about
    1½ pints for an adult, ½ pint for a child
Lotion thermometer
Large bowl containing enema apparatus :
    Large glass funnel
    Length of tubing
    Glass connection
    Catheter No. 10 to 12 for an adult
    Catheter No. 6 to 8 for a child
    Tubing clip
Large receiver for used catheter

A drink of water should be at hand in case the patient feels faint after the enema is given, also a warmed bedpan and cover, with toilet paper or tow.

Method. Bring the covered tray to the bedside and place the bedpan within reach.

Turn back the bedclothes, leaving the patient covered with a blanket.

Place the patient, if possible, in the *left lateral* position (Fig. 7, p. 62), with the knees bent and the buttocks well to the edge of the bed, otherwise in the dorsal position.

Arrange the plastic square and towel under the patient to protect the bed.

Expel air from the apparatus by running a little of the enema solution through it and pinching the tubing with the clip before the funnel is quite empty.

Lubricate the end of the catheter and insert into the rectum for 3 or 4 inches.

Hold the funnel about a foot above the buttocks and allow about 5 minutes for the fluid to run in.

Withdraw the catheter gently before the funnel is quite empty and encourage the patient to hold the fluid for 2 or 3 minutes.

Place the patient on the bedpan, supporting him if necessary and giving him a drink if he feels faint.

When removing the bedpan see that the patient is left quite clean and comfortable.

The result of the enema must not be emptied away until the nurse has made sure that it will not be necessary to save it for sister's or doctor's inspection.

If the solution has not been returned, the nurse must report the matter at once to the sister in charge of the ward, so that the enema solution may be syphoned back.

The apparatus must be washed and the catheter cleaned and boiled.

Starch and opium enema. 15 to 30 minims of opium in 2 to 4 ounces of liquid starch may be ordered to check diarrhoea.

A *suppository* is a solid, cone-shaped preparation containing, or made of, a substance which will give a bowel action without the delay of an aperient or the discomfort of an enema. For these reasons they are used frequently. Dulcolax and glycerin are the best known.

The patient is asked to lie on her left side, and the nurse, wearing a rubber glove, dips the suppository into a bowl of warm water and inserts it gently into the rectum for a few inches. It should melt and give a good bowel action within half an hour.

RECTAL WASHOUT

This may be ordered to check diarrhoea, or to empty the bowel before a special examination or operation on the rectum.

The trolley should contain:

Plastic sheet and cotton square to place under the patient's buttocks
Two large jugs containing hot water. From 4 to 8 pints may be needed
A jug for giving the washout at 38° C (100° F)
Lotion thermometer
Petroleum jelly
Gallipot containing a few swabs or pieces of old linen

The lower shelf of the trolley should contain:

A waterproof sheet to protect the floor
Bucket for the returned fluid
Bowl for used towels
Receiver for used swabs
Large receiver for used rectal tube
The method is the same as that employed in giving an enema but the lotion ordered is slowly run into the bowel at the correct temperature and syphoned back, i.e. the fluid is poured into the funnel and before the funnel is quite empty, it is turned upside down over the bucket. The procedure is repeated until the returned fluid is quite clear. Anything unusual must be reported to the sister or nurse in charge of the ward.

PASSING A FLATUS TUBE

A flatus tube is a long rubber tube which differs from a catheter in that it has an opening at the extreme end instead of an eye at the side. It may be inserted into the rectum and left in position for a short time in order to relieve abdominal distension due to the accumulation of gas in the lower bowel, often after an abdominal operation.

The tube is softened by placing it in a bowl of warm water, the air is expelled, the end is lubricated with petroleum jelly and inserted into the rectum for 3 or 4 inches, and the free end is kept under the water.

Bubbles in the water are an indication that flatus is being passed.

The flatus tube may be attached to a length of tubing and a glass funnel, because this makes it easier to expel air from the tube.

After the patient has had some relief, leave him comfortable and clear away.

If possible, the patient should lie in the *left lateral* position (Fig. 7).

GIVING A RECTAL SALINE

This may be ordered when a patient is not taking sufficient nourishment by mouth, or when for some reason, the stomach must have rest, or when the body has lost much fluid, by sweating, vomiting and diarrhoea, haemorrhage, or from skin wounds, such as burns.

Normal saline is prepared by adding one teaspoonful of salt to a pint of water. This must be heated to 38° C (100° F) so as to reach the tissues at body temperature. Glucose, two teaspoonfuls to a pint, may sometimes be added.

Before the saline is given, the bowel and bladder must be empty, and where the patient is suffering from flatulence, a flatus tube should be passed, otherwise the saline will not be retained.

The same articles are needed as for an enema, but a smaller catheter will be used, and a smaller funnel to avoid cooling the saline.

The method of giving a saline is similar to that employed for an enema, but the funnel must be held only slightly higher than the patient's buttocks so that the fluid may run in *very* slowly, about twenty minutes being taken to allow time for it to be absorbed. If a continuous saline is to be given, which is of much more value, the fluid is obtained from the dispensary in a special flask, and hung on a 'drip' stand. The rubber tubing is attached to a drip connection and the saline is allowed to enter the rectum one drop at a time for 24 hours or longer.

14

Helping the Doctor

A good deal of a nurse's work consists of preparing the articles that a doctor will need when he comes to examine a patient or to do some treatment in the ward.

She should have everything neatly arranged on a tray or trolley, the curtains drawn round the bed, the patient resting quietly in the correct position, knowing what is expected of him and with some idea of what the examination or treatment will be.

When the doctor arrives, the nurse will stand quietly by, ready to hand him anything he requires or she may stand by the patient ready to turn or lift him as needed.

In many hospitals new sets of apparatus or instruments for procedures described below will be obtained ready packed from the Central Sterile Supply department, but the nurse should learn what each contains.

Examination of the Rectum

An examination of the rectum may be made by the doctor in order to discover whether a patient is suffering from:

Enlarged prostate gland	Pelvic abscesses
Haemorrhoids	Diseases of the uterus
Carcinoma of the rectum	Appendicitis, etc

She must arrange the patient in the *left lateral* position (Fig. 7), where this is possible, and turn down the bedclothes, leaving the patient covered with a blanket.

Helping the Doctor

The bowel and bladder must be empty and the part clean.

Required for a rectal examination:

Plastic square and towel in receiver
Receiver containing right-hand rubber, or plastic gloves or
    finger stalls
Receiver for used finger stalls
French chalk in dredger
Petroleum jelly
Swabs or pieces of old linen in gallipot
Small receiver for used swabs

If required to do so by the doctor, the nurse may put out a rectal speculum and a bell light or torch.

Examination of the Vagina

A doctor may require to make an examination of the vagina to discover whether a patient has any abnormal condition of the uterus or vagina.

For such an examination the nurse must see that the bowel and bladder are empty and the patient is perfectly clean, that everything needed during the examination is rendered absolutely sterile, and that provision is made for the surgeon to wash his hands.

Articles required for examination of the vagina:

Plastic square
Bowl containing sterile dressing towels, swabs and pads
Bowl for used towels
Receiver for used swabs
Receiver containing sterile gloves in packet
French chalk
Lubricant, e.g. Dettol cream
Bowl of lotion, antiseptic as ordered
Sterile dressing forceps
Receiver for used instruments
Vaginal speculum

Bell lamp or torch
Bowl of sterile water

Examination of the Throat, Nose and Ear

Before any condition of the throat can be treated, the doctor will require to make an examination, and for this the nurse must prepare:

A head mirror
Torch
Plastic cape and towel to be placed around the patient's neck
Wooden spatulae
Tongue depressor
Sponge-holding forceps, or probes tipped with sterile wool
(if the throat may require painting or in case a specimen is to be sent to the laboratory)
Culture tubes
Form for pathological investigation
Throat mirrors
Swabs and folded pieces of gauze
Receiver for used swabs
Bowl of antiseptic for used mirrors
Spirit lamp to warm the mirrors so that they do not steam over
Matches
Cocaine or other local anaesthetic, throat spray (if ordered)
Mouth wash
Receiver
Towel

If the nose and ears are to be examined at the same time, as is usual, the following should be added:

Aural and nasal specula
Nasal forceps
Auriscope

All these instruments are kept together as a set.

The patient faces the light with his head supported by the nurse. Remove any dentures.

Lumbar Puncture

The nurse may be called upon to help when a doctor is going to perform this investigation. She will see him insert a special needle into the lower part of the back and draw off some of the cerebrospinal fluid which lies between the coverings of the spinal cord.

She will remember that the cord itself ends at the level of the first lumbar vertebra, therefore the puncture will be made lower than this so that the delicate nerves are not injured.

She will prepare a trolley containing:

Sterile swabs and towels
Small gauze dressing
Plastic square
Bowls and receivers
Lotion to clean the skin (e.g. cetrimide, ether or spirit)
Hypodermic syringe and needles
Local anaesthetic
Sterile test tubes and laboratory forms
Collodion to seal the wound
Forceps and scissors
Two or three special lumbar puncture needles, manometer and rubber tubing to attach it. (This is to record the pressure when the fluid comes out.)

This treatment is done to find out whether the patient has any germs such as meningococci or streptococci in his cerebrospinal fluid, or the presence of blood and a raised pressure may indicate a tumour in the brain or cord.

Sometimes lumbar puncture is done to give a spinal anaesthetic, or to give a drug such as streptomycin or penicillin.

Before the doctor comes the nurse will place the patient in the left lateral position with the head and shoulders bent over as far as possible, the buttocks to the edge of the bed.

Afterwards the patient must be nursed flat for a few hours as he may suffer from a severe headache.

The doctor may also order the foot of the bed to be raised on blocks.

Blood Transfusion and Blood Grouping

When a patient has lost a lot of blood, the only thing which may save his life is a blood transfusion, which means the giving of another person's blood. However, although all blood, even that of animals, contains the same basic things, there are certain differences that are extremely important. We now know that if a patient receives blood that does not mix properly with his own, there can be terrible consequences, and the person will be worse off than if he had not received any blood at all. Indeed transfusing the wrong type of blood may lead to the death of the patient.

It has been found that human blood falls into four groups, called simply enough A, B, AB and O, and everyone's blood belongs to one or other of these groups. Now the red blood cells are very delicate little things, and they are most sensitive to the plasma they live in. They are all right in their own plasma, but if a few red cells were put, say, into a drop of plasma from a horse, they would all clump together and in a few minutes break up and be no further use. Similarly if human blood of different groups is mixed, the red blood cells may form clumps, instead of moving freely.

It is essential therefore, before carrying out a transfusion, to find out to which group the patient's blood belongs and to provide blood that is suitable for him.

People with Group AB blood can receive blood from any group but can give blood only to Group AB.

People with Group A blood can receive blood from Groups A and O but can give blood only to Groups AB and A.

People with Group B blood can receive blood from Groups B and O but can give blood only to Groups AB and B.

People with Group O blood can receive blood only from Group O but can give blood to all groups.

The Group O people therefore are in the happy position of

being able to give their blood to anyone, if they are good enough to become donors — in fact they are called 'universal donors', and are rather rare and sought after people. The Group AB people are lucky too, on their own account, as *they* can receive blood from anyone, so are called 'universal recipients'.

So now you will see why it is so important for the blood bottles to be checked and rechecked before blood is given in transfusion. The right blood will give Life—the wrong one, Death.

Intravenous injections and blood transfusions are always given by the doctor, but the nurse will be called upon to prepare the apparatus and to assist. She will prepare a trolley containing:

Sterile swabs and gauze dressings in bowls
Receivers for used swabs and instruments
Sterile towels. Spirit for cleaning the skin
Local anaesthetic, hypodermic syringe and needles
A 2 ml. (or 10 ml. or 20 ml.) syringe and the drug to be given
A tourniquet or sphygmomanometer
A scalpel
One toothed and one plain dissecting forceps
One pair fine scissors
Two pairs fine artery forceps
One aneurysm needle
Intravenous cannula
Suture thread for tying in the cannula
Two curved needles and skin suture thread
One sterile giving set
A 'drip' stand will be placed by the bed if a continuous drip is contemplated. If blood is to be given, this will be fetched as ordered, or brought by the doctor. If saline is to be given it will be fetched already prepared from the dispensary.

15

Preventing Infection

A wound is an opening into the skin or any other covering of the body or its organs. It may come about by accident, or be made on purpose by a surgeon. A wound may be caused by cuts, laceration (tearing), by burns or friction, by stabbing, by the entry by force of a foreign body, and even a small thing like a prick can be called a wound.

Once an opening has been made, bacteria (germs) can find their way in and cause inflammation and sepsis unless we are very careful.

Infection

Infection is the entry of disease-producing bacteria into the body, where they develop and multiply and give off poisons known as toxins, which cause many of the symptoms of disease.

Bacteria are present everywhere in the air, especially if it contains dust, in unpurified water, in soil, in food and in milk, in the human throat, mouth, and skin, especially the nails.

They need food, heat, moisture and darkness, and find these in the human body, which they enter:

1. By inhalation, i.e. through the air breathed into the lungs.
2. By ingestion, i.e. the taking of infected food, milk or water into the digestive tract.

3. By inoculation, i.e. through a cut or prick in the surface of the skin or mucous membrane.

Inflammation

Inflammation is the reaction of the tissues to injury or infection.

The signs and symptoms of inflammation are:

Redness—heat—swelling—pain—loss of function, and general malaise, or a feeling of illness, with
    A rise of temperature, and possibly
    A rigor
    Headache
    Hot dry skin
    Constipation, concentrated scanty urine

Inflammation may end uneventfully if the lymphatic vessels and glands are able to remove the poison causing the disturbance.

If they are not able to do their work properly, part of the products of inflammation may be converted into fibrous tissue, or suppuration may occur and even death of the part.

TERMS USED IN CONNECTION WITH INFLAMMATION

Suppuration, the formation of pus.

Ulcer, the death of tissue occurring on a free surface.

Gangrene, the death of an organ or part.

Abscess, a collection of pus surrounded by a wall of living tissue.

Cellulitis, spreading inflammation of the cellular tissue.

Toxaemia, a state of blood poisoning due to the presence in the blood stream of toxins (poisons) from a wound.

Septicaemia, a state of blood poisoning due to the presence in the blood stream of bacteria as well as their toxins.

Healing takes place by the formation of new tissue, fibrous and tough. When there is no sepsis and the edges of the wound are brought neatly together and held there by stitches or strapping for a few days, a new row of cells soon forms, over which the skin grows, and only a thin line is seen. This is called healing by first intention.

Sometimes the wound is too big or deep for the edges to come together, especially if there has been sepsis. In this case a great many new cells are required, and tiny blood vessels branch out from nearby capillaries to feed them as they grow up, layer by layer. This flesh is called granulation tissue, and takes longer to heal. This is healing by second intention. It may leave quite a big scar, on which no hair will grow.

In the early days of surgery, no attention was paid to what we now call surgical cleanliness, but when the great French chemist, Louis Pasteur, proved that some diseases were due to germs, and that germs also caused wounds to become septic, it became customary, by using strong disinfectants like carbolic on wounds, to try to kill these germs before they entered the body.

It was found, however, that disinfectants burnt and injured the tissues, so that the patient was not much better off. This fact led to the discovery that if everything in contact with a wound could be kept free from germs, the wound would not become septic and these harmful disinfectants would be unnecessary.

Notice the difference between these words:

A disinfectant is something strong enough to kill bacteria.

An antiseptic is not so powerful, but it can stop bacteria from multiplying even if it does not kill the ones already present.

Asepsis means a state of being completely free from bacteria.

In modern surgical work, *antiseptics* are used to prepare the patient's skin for operation. *Asepsis* is attained by rendering all articles used during the operation, e.g. dressings, instruments, etc., free from germs by sterilizing them by steam under pressure or by boiling.

Surgical cleanliness therefore means much more than ordinary cleanliness. It means complete absence of those bacteria which are normally present on the skin and which could enter a wound and cause infection.

Disinfection

Disinfection is the process of rendering an article free from germs by means of:

Exposure to sunlight. The ultra-violet rays of the sun are effective in killing germs.

Sterilizing by steam under pressure for a given time.

Boiling for 5 minutes will kill all organisms. Used for glass syringes, test tubes and laboratory apparatus.

Dry heat. The articles are exposed to a temperature of 113° C (300° F) for one hour.

Immersion in certain disinfectants

All disinfectants used externally should be kept in coloured, ridged bottles so as to be recognized both by sight and by touch. They should always be put away in a safe place after use and kept under lock and key.

This applies also to urine testing reagents.

There are now many disinfectants, and one which is used in one hospital may be unknown in another. This does not mean that one is therefore better than another. The people who buy supplies like to try out different things, and when they find one which is suitable they may not find any reason to change, especially as all drugs, medicines, lotions, disinfectants, etc, are expensive. For this reason, very few disinfectants and their strengths are given in this book. Figures can be very confusing.

FIND OUT what is in use in your ward or hospital. The strength at which to use it will either be on the bottle or in directions in every ward. IF IN DOUBT—ASK.

NEVER be tempted to use these substances in greater strengths than the directions say. To do so is wasteful and may be dangerous. A germ can only die once!

SOME OF THE ANTISEPTICS AND DISINFECTANTS IN COMMON
USE

Boracic lotion is a mild, non-irritating lotion used chiefly for
bathing sore eyes.

Bradosol is a detergent (grease removing) and antiseptic
agent, used for cleaning the skin, or for instruments, bowls, etc.

Carbolic acid (phenol) is still used for disinfecting stools, linen,
etc. Very effective but can burn the skin.

Cetavlon or *centrimide* has a similar action to Bradosol.

Eusol is a lotion made from lime and boracic. Used for washing out septic wounds, or for hot soaks for septic fingers, etc.

Hibitane is much used today, because it is a good disinfectant
yet does not hurt the tissues.

Iodine is made from seaweed. It is rarely used now as some
people are very sensitive to it, and may get a rash, so NEVER
use it if a patient tells you he does not like it. Find out from
sister what else can be used for the purpose.

Izal and *Jeyes Fluid* are strong, soapy solutions of coal tar.
They are used only for disinfecting lavatories, sluices, and
brushes used there.

Lysol and *Sudol* are sometimes used for cleaning baths, or for
disinfecting excreta or bedpans. They are dangerous because
they can burn the hands, so must not be allowed to touch the
skin.

Milton is useful and safe. It is much used for sterilizing
babies' feeding bottles in a 1 in 80 solution.

Roccal is another detergent and disinfecting agent. It is blue
in colour and does not stain. It is used for many purposes, from
sterilizing thermometers and instruments to preparing the skin
before operation.

Savlon concentrate is similar to Roccal, and is used for general
antiseptic purposes.

THE PREPARATION OF LOTIONS

Many lotions are made double strength, so need diluting with
an equal volume of water. Others are sent to the wards in strong

solutions, and have to be diluted. This must always be done with great care, and the dilution should be worked out on paper first.

The easiest way to do this is to take the strength of the solution which you HAVE, and divide it by the figure you WANT, so:

EXAMPLE: *Make up a pint of* 1:80 *from a strength of* 1:20.
Divide 80 by 20, which gives 4 parts.
Take a fourth of a pint, i.e. 5 ounces of 1:20 and three fourths of water, i.e. 15 ounces.
This gives 20 ounces of the required lotion:

$$\text{or} \quad \frac{\text{HAVE} \quad 20:}{\text{WANT} \quad 80:}$$

ANSWER is the amount of stock to be used. The rest is water.

Normal saline is made by adding one drachm of common salt to one pint of water, or two tablets of sodium chloride, i.e. 80 grains. This quantity is equal to the amount of salt in the blood and body tissues.

As a rule, saline is made double strength, i.e. one drachm to half a pint of water, so that it can be diluted for use by adding an equal quantity of hot, sterile water.

THE CLEANING AND STERILIZATION OF ARTICLES IN COMMON USE

Anything which contains protein 'sets' if you put it in hot water. (Think of the white of an egg, which is all protein.) So since blood, pus, and all excreta from the body contain protein, always wash first in cold water anything which may have come in contact with any of these things.

Dressings, waterproof sheeting and towels, enclosed in special drums or packets, are sterilized in an autoclave by means of steam at a high pressure.

Gloves which are not of the disposable type, are rinsed in cold water after use then washed in hot soapy water inside and out.

They can be boiled for 3 minutes. They should then be drained, tested for holes, dried, and put in pairs, a left with a right, in their correct sizes, i.e. an 8 with an 8, a 6½ with a 6½. The cuffs are turned up, both surfaces of the gloves are dusted with special powder, and they are sent to be autoclaved.

Rubber catheters and rubber tubing, etc. After use catheters must always be washed in warm soapy water, rinsed and held under the tap to cleanse through the eye. If the eye is blocked it must be cleaned out with a syringe.

A solution of bicarbonate of soda will remove pus from drainage tubes.

After cleansing, rubber catheters and rubber tubing should be boiled in plain water for 5 minutes and plunged in cold, sterile water to restore the tone of the rubber.

Elastic gum catheters should be placed dry in a special formalin cabinet on perforated trays for 24 hours. They may also be immersed in biniodide of mercury 1:1,000 for 30 minutes. In emergency they can be wrapped in lint and boiled, but for 2 minutes only, longer boiling will soften them and make them useless.

They must always be rinsed in plain sterile water before use.

Bougies, which resemble catheters except that they have no eye, are treated in the same way.

Syringes which are not of the disposable type should be rinsed in cold water after use, taken to pieces, then washed, and boiled in plain water for 5 minutes if they are combined glass and metal. Some syringes are made entirely of glass and are sterilized by dry heat at a syringe centre. In either case, the parts must be wrapped up very carefully to avoid breakage.

Syringes may be stored in surgical spirit and rinsed before use in cold sterile water, and in some cases distilled water, but forceps must be used when handling them. Before a syringe is put together again, see that it is quite cold, otherwise it may break, as glass and metal cool at different rates.

Glass must be wrapped in old linen or lint and placed in cold water in a container to prevent breakage. It must be brought slowly to the boil, boiled for 5 minutes and cooled slowly.

Enamelware should be thoroughly cleaned and rinsed after use then sterilized by boiling for 5 minutes in a large bowl sterilizer or a pail.

Sharp cutting instruments, knives and needles should be cleaned and sterilized by placing in disinfectant such as Cetavlon or Hibitane for 3 minutes or they may be wrapped in lint and boiled for 2 minutes, then placed in spirit until required. Before use, the instruments must be well rinsed in cold, sterile water.

THE CARE AND DISINFECTION OF INSTRUMENTS

After use, instruments must be opened or taken apart and scrubbed with a nail brush in cold water, then in warm, soapy water, then rinsed, and boiled for 5 minutes.

A piece of lint should be placed over the bottom of the sterilizer to prevent spotting, and soda, a drachm to the pint, added to increase the boiling point.

Immerse the instruments when the water is boiling, as this expels the air and prevents rusting.

If for use immediately place dry on a sterile tray.

Instruments not required immediately should be dried, the joints should be smeared with petroleum jelly and they should be put away in an airtight cupboard.

Many hospitals now have a Central Sterile Supply Department (CSSD). Instruments, dressings and other equipment are sent to the wards in packs, already sterilized. Much of the equipment is of the disposable type, e.g. gloves, catheters, syringes, and is thrown away after use. The rest is returned to the CSSD to be resterilized. No sterilizing is carried out in the wards.

This is an invaluable service because it enables the nurse to spend much more time with the patients, but until it is available in all hospitals it will be necessary for her to know how to sterilize equipment in the ward.

How Infection is Spread

Once infection has gained a hold in a person it can be passed on to other people in the following ways:

1. Direct contact with a diseased person or with the discharges from his body, e.g. the venereal diseases.
2. Fomites, i.e. articles such as clothing, toys, crockery, etc, used by the patient, e.g. measles.
3. Droplet infection, when the germs are conveyed by coughing or sneezing, e.g. influenza, colds.
4. Airborne infection, when germs are blown about by dust, e.g. dried sputum containing tubercle bacilli.
5. Carriers, i.e. people who hold in their bodies the germs of a disease without suffering from it themselves, or after recovery from it; e.g. typhoid bacilli may be passed in the stool; streptococci are often found in the nose and throat of apparently healthy people.
6. Flies which may carry any infection on their legs and feet. Other insects such as fleas, bugs, and lice may carry bacteria.
7. Water, which is sometimes infected by typhoid, paratyphoid and dysentery organisms.
8. Milk, which may also be responsible for outbreaks of any of these diseases or may carry living tubercle bacilli.
9. Food, which may become contaminated by certain organisms, occasionally resulting in food poisoning. The most commonly affected foods are meat pies, sausages, and meat pastes.

Infectious diseases are always regarded as a grave public danger. They may occur in various forms.

A sporadic outbreak is one where there is a limited number of widely separated people affected.

An endemic outbreak is where a disease occurs constantly in one area over a long period of time, e.g. plague is endemic to India.

An epidemic refers to a large number of cases occurring in one
area within a limited period.

Prevention of the Spread of Infection in the Community

All cases of infectious disease must be notified to the Medical
Officer of Health, who will take steps to prevent the infection
from spreading by:
1. Tracing the source of the infection and removing it.
2. Seeing that those who have been in contact with the
   infected person are given treatment and kept apart from
   other people until all danger of further infection has
   passed.

The patient is best nursed in an isolation hospital, or barrier
nursed in a general one.

Barrier nursing means putting a barrier between the infected
patient and the rest of the ward, and taking precautions to see
that germs from the patient do not cross the barrier.

The barrier has no power to prevent germs from spreading.
It is simply a reminder to the nurse that these precautions
must always be taken when nursing the infected patient. In
an open ward the barrier is usually a screen at the end of the
patient's bed, the bed itself being placed in a corner of the ward
away from other patients.

Nurses can carry infection on their uniforms from one
patient to another, therefore gowns are always worn over
uniforms when attending to the patient. Masks are worn if
the patient's illness is of the kind which spreads by droplet
infection from his nose and mouth.

Gowns are put on, taken off and hung up in such a way that
the 'clean' inside is protected.

The nurse must wash her hands thoroughly *after* attending
to the patient, or touching anything inside the barrier, and
before she touches anything 'clean'.

As far as possible disposable equipment is used. All articles
which cannot be burnt after use are carefully sterilized, either
by boiling or by soaking in disinfectant.

Other precautionary measures against infection are immunization against diseases such as diphtheria and scarlet fever, vaccination against smallpox, poliomyelitis, colds and whooping cough, and the injection of serum to guard against diseases such as measles.

Immunity

Immunity is a condition in which the body is able to resist certain diseases.

Whenever germs enter the body, white cells known as *phagocytes* multiply in the blood stream to deal with them and special substances known as antibodies are produced.

Immunity may be *inherited* when it is spoken of as *natural immunity,* thus, a breast-fed baby will inherit its mother's immunity to some diseases, at least for the first few months of its life, by which time it will be making its own antibodies; immunity may also be *acquired*.

Acquired immunity may be *active* or *passive*.

Active immunity is obtained by stimulating the tissue cells of the body to produce their own antibodies by:

1. Having an attack of the disease.
2. Inoculating the patient with a vaccine, i.e. to give the patient a very mild form of the disease and cause his body to manufacture immunizing substances.

   This is done in the case of smallpox and poliomyelitis.

Passive immunity is obtained by the introduction of antitoxins, e.g. in the case of diphtheria and measles.

Antitoxic sera are prepared by inoculating an animal with increasingly large doses of an organism so that in time it becomes immunized. The blood is then drawn from a vein, and the serum, loaded with antibodies, is injected into a patient, e.g. horse serum in the case of a patient suffering from diphtheria or tetanus.

Serum from the blood of those who have had the disease can be given to protect children against the commoner infections such as measles. That of a patient or of any suitable adult may be used.

Stock vaccines are prepared from any suitable source and kept ready for use, e.g. the now famous Salk vaccine against polio-myelitis.

Cross Infection

Hospitals are full to overflowing with germs. Not only the relatively mild germs which we all encounter everywhere, but virulent highly dangerous ones as well. It is quite possible for a patient to come into hospital for some simple form of treatment and while there to pick up an infection which makes him seriously ill.

This passing of germs from one patient to another is called cross infection. It is so widespread that the Minister of Health has recommended every hospital to have a Control of Infection Officer.

Infection spreads in hospital through the same channels as it does in the community (p. 138). But the three most important ways are by people's mouths, noses and hands.

Mr A. uses a bedpan and you forget to give him a bowl to wash his hands. There are many germs in the colon and now some of them are on Mr A.'s *hands*. Mr A. has a drainage tube in his side and it feels uncomfortable so he pulls at the dressing to ease it. Now the germs are on the *dressing*. You come along to change his dressing and forget to wash your hands after removing the bandage. Now the germs are on your *hands* and on the *trolley*. You don't bother to clean the trolley before you go on to the next patient and now the germs are free, out of control in the open *ward,* going from patient to patient.

Every time Mr B. coughs a fine spray of germs flies out of his mouth and settles on his bedclothes. It dries quickly and when you come to make his bed the dried germs are tossed into the air. Some of them settle on the book which Mr C. has put on his bedtable. Mr C. picks his book up and starts reading. Becoming absorbed in the story he absentmindedly chews his thumbnail—and Mr B's germs have found a new home.

Nurse D. comes on duty with a nasty cold. She gives her nose a good blow, stuffs her hanky in her pocket and hurries off to help sister serve lunch. By now you know how the story goes on—germs on every plate, all the way round the ward in ten minutes flat.

PREVENTION OF CROSS INFECTION

Cross infection can be prevented if you follow a few simple rules of cleanliness for yourself, the patient and the ward.

For yourself:

1. Wash your hands *before* touching food, or sterile articles and sterile equipment.
2. Wash your hands *after* you have touched infected material, such as bedpans, urinals, dressings, specimens, and after going to the lavatory.
3. Keep your nails short and clean.
4. If you have a cold, a sore throat, a septic finger, or any other infection, report it to sister at once.

For the patient:

1. See that patients wash their hands after going to the lavatory or using a bedpan.
2. Be scrupulous in observing all the rules of asepsis when you are carrying out a sterile procedure for the patient.

For the ward:

1. Keep the ward as well aired as you can without causing draughts. If you go outside the ward for a few minutes and then come back again you will be able to tell as you walk through the door whether the ward smells fresh or not.
2. When you make beds do so with as little disturbance as possible so that germs are not scattered into the air.

3. Use cotton blankets in place of woollen, because they can be boiled frequently.

4. Wait for at least an hour after bedmaking and ward cleaning has finished before doing dressings. This gives time for the germ-laden dust to settle.

5. See that dirty dressings and dirty linen are put straight into the special containers provided, and are not left open to the air.

6. Use paper towels in kitchen and wash room, and paper handkerchiefs.

Because we cannot see the germs around us it is hard to believe that they are really there, but during your training you will be shown some under a microscope and then you will realize how important these rules are—not only for the patient's sake, but for your own as well.

16

Working in a Surgical Ward

You will find that operations will fall into five main classes:
  1. *Emergency*. These are the cases that must be operated on at once to save life, even if there is no time to undress or prepare the patient in any way. These include cases where the patient is bleeding uncontrollably, e.g. ruptured ectopic (Fallopian) tube, ruptured spleen, accident cases where an artery is severed.
  2. *Urgency*. These are cases which need surgery very quickly, but there is an hour or two in which to give a blood transfusion, or treat for shock, or replace lost fluids, e.g. perforated gastric ulcer, strangulated hernia.
  3. *Necessity*. This means the operation really must be done if the patient is ever to live a normal life again. This class includes those done for patients with cancer, like amputation of the breast, or removal of causes of sepsis, like appendicectomy, or amputations of limbs when gangrene has started, and many others. This is perhaps the biggest group.
  4. *Expediency*. This means, 'It really ought to be done—you will be much better afterwards'. This group includes things like the operation to cure a hernia (rupture), or removal of tonsils after many septic throats, while a great many gynaecological operations come into this class, like repairs after childbirth.

5. The rest may be called operations of *choice*. You may wonder how anyone can choose to have an operation—it seems an odd thing to *want*, but there are many conditions which, though not dangerous, or even painful, may still cause a lot of misery in daily life by making people seem odd, or not able to do as much as their companions, yet which can be put right or greatly improved. Many of these are 'chosen' for children by their parents—the operation to cure squinting eyes, or the repair of a cleft palate, while many orthopaedic operations for straightening deformities, etc., come into this class, and many of the plastic operations for improving the appearance of the face or hands after accidents like burns.

Preparation of the Patient for Operation

Where possible a patient is admitted to hospital a few days before the operation so that he may have sufficient rest and so that any special investigations and preparations which the doctor considers necessary may be made without difficulty. In all cases where an anaesthetic is to be given, consent for operation must be obtained from the patient or his next of kin. An identification bracelet is attached to his wrist giving his name and hospital number.

The enrolled nurse will help the sister or nurse in charge of the ward by carrying out her duties quickly and quietly and by her calm manner she will give confidence to the patient before and during his ordeal.

As a rule, an aperient is ordered two nights before, and an enema may be ordered on the morning of the operation.

The patient has a bath and the skin is shaved and prepared aseptically the day before and again on the morning of the operation, and the area may be covered with a sterile towel and bandage.

Before an operation it is necessary to build up a store of sugar in the liver to counteract the effects of the anaesthetic, therefore the surgeon may order plenty of fluids containing glucose, a drachm to a pint on the previous day. Barley sugar may be ordered as an alternative in the case of a child. Sometimes extra vitamins will be given in tablet form. The blood will be tested for its group, in case a transfusion is needed later.

If the operation is in the morning, the patient usually has a light breakfast of tea and toast, but if it is in the afternoon he may also have light nourishment in the middle of the morning. In all cases, however, *exact* instructions will be given by the surgeon and the nurse must obey them.

The patient is dressed in a warm, open backed gown and theatre cap and long woollen socks are pulled on over his feet.

Dentures are removed, and all jewellery except a wedding ring. A bedpan or urinal is given. In some operations on the pelvic organs a catheter may have to be passed, and left in position with a spigot to block the open end.

If urine has not been passed in sufficient quantity, the surgeon must be informed, as it may be necessary for the patient to be catheterized.

The patient is then placed on the trolley, warmly covered up, and the drug ordered is given by the nurse.

At the appointed time he is taken to the operating theatre, and the nurse accompanying him takes with her a vomit bowl and towel, and instruments which may be needed after the operation. These are sponge-holding forceps with gauze swab in place, tongue forceps and mouth gag. She also takes any notes and films which the surgeon may need.

The nurse who goes with the patient to theatre must know his full name, the operation he is to have, what premedication has been given to him, and when he last had anything to eat or drink.

She is personally responsible for seeing that the details on the notes and films correspond with those on his identification bracelet.

The enrolled nurse will help the sister or nurse in charge of the ward by carrying out her duties quickly and quietly in a calm manner. By using her imagination she can give support and confidence to the patient before and during his ordeal.

A bedpan is a most awkward and uncomfortable thing to manage, even if you are quite well. It can be misery for a patient who meets it for the first time when he is weak and in pain. After his operation the patient may have to use one for some time. He will find it so much easier if you get him to practise for a couple of days before the operation. Explain why you are suggesting this and he will probably be only too pleased to do as you say.

Try to remember that although the pre-operative routine of aperient, enema, bath, shave, is commonplace to you it is all strange to the patient. He doesn't understand the need for it and each unexpected procedure just adds to his apprehension. Tell him beforehand that he will be having an enema, or that he will be shaved, and explain briefly why it is necessary. To start shaving a woman between her legs without warning or explanation is thoroughly bad nursing, and the nurse who can do such a thing simply shows what little human understanding she has.

Patients naturally have fears about operations. Try to find out what worries them. Questions about the outcome of the operation you must refer to sister or the doctor, but there are often things which you, yourself, can answer. For example, many patients are afraid that the surgeon will start operating before they are really unconscious. It helps a lot if you tell them that the anaesthetic is given in a room outside the theatre, and that the anaesthetist will not let a patient be taken into theatre until he is right under.

If you have had an operation yourself you will know how they are feeling. If not, just get your imagination to work.

Treatment of the Patient After the Operation

While the patient is in the theatre the bed is prepared according to the nature of the operation, and any extra articles which may be needed after the patient has recovered from the anaesthetic must be placed in readiness because he must not be left until consciousness has been regained.

Articles which may be needed include:

> Recovery tray with mouth gag, tongue forceps, sponge
>   holders, dry and wet swabs, vomit bowl and towel
> Extra pillows, waterproof sheeting, and drawsheets
> Backrest
> Sandbags
> Air ring
> Cradles
> Blocks
> Stand for drip apparatus

Many nurses and porters find it difficult to move a patient
from a stretcher to a bed. Here is a good method.

Move the locker and any equipment away from the side of the
bed.

Place the head of the stretcher *at right angles to the foot of the
bed.*

Three people stand on the side of the stretcher nearest to the
bed.

One takes the patient's head and shoulders, one his hips and
the third his legs.

All three bend their knees and slip their arms well under the
patient, getting a really firm grip.

Moving together they roll him towards them, lift him up,
and turn towards the bed.

Bending again from the knees they lower him gently on to the
bed.

The person carrying his head and shoulders should be careful
to see that his head is supported throughout.

The *position of the patient* after return from the theatre is
semi-prone, if possible, otherwise on his side, with his knees
bent and his head flat on the bed with no pillow.

A plastic square and towel should be placed under the chin.

Afterwards the position will be according to the wishes of the
surgeon, e.g. a patient who has had an operation on the abdomen
with drainage may be propped up in Fowler's position.

It may be necessary to raise the foot of the bed on blocks.

The nurse must watch for signs of shock, and be ready to treat it according to the way she has been taught at her hospital. Protect the patient from draughts, but see that he is not over-heated, and report his condition to the nurse in charge.

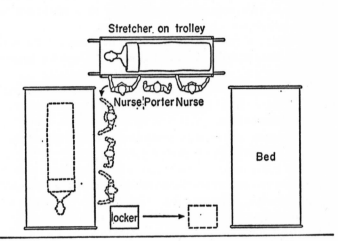

FIG. 11. MOVING A PATIENT FROM A STRETCHER TO A BED

The pulse must be recorded every 15 minutes, and any weakening or increase in rate be reported at once. The nurse must note any signs of increasing *pallor* or *blueness*.

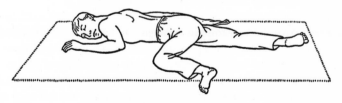

FIG. 12. THE SEMI-PRONE POSITION

149

If any difficulty occurs in breathing she must clear the patient's throat of mucus, hold his jaw forward to open his airway and call sister at once.

The number of times vomiting occurs must be noted and the nature of the vomit. Report any persistent vomiting and when retching occurs, support the wound by pressure with the hand upon it. A mouth gag may be used to keep the patient's mouth open if he is vomiting while still unconscious. Fortunately vomiting is rare with the improvement in anaesthetics and surgical techniques.

The wound should not be disturbed or dressed without the orders of the surgeon, but a watch must be kept for haemorrhage.

When a patient complains of pain, see that he is comfortably placed in bed and that the bandages are not too tight and report the complaint to sister.

A hypodermic tray must be ready in case a drug is ordered for the relief of pain or in the case of collapse.

Except in gastric cases, fluids may as a rule be given as soon as the patient recovers from the anaesthetic, at first in sips only. Unless vomiting is severe, light diet will soon be given after which there is a gradual return to normal diet.

Aperients are given only when ordered by the doctor. As a rule, they are ordered the third night after operation. If an aperient is not successful, an enema may be ordered to be given eight hours later.

Urine. Note the quantity and colour of the urine, the presence of any abnormalities and whether there is retention which must be treated by external methods first. Catheterization should not be done until all these have failed (p. 115).

Patients are not allowed to get up after an operation until the surgeon gives permission but it is usual to let them sit out of bed for a short time about 24 to 48 hours after most operations. This movement helps to prevent chest complications and the clotting of blood in the leg veins. It also has a cheering effect on the patient and makes him feel he is already on the road to recovery.

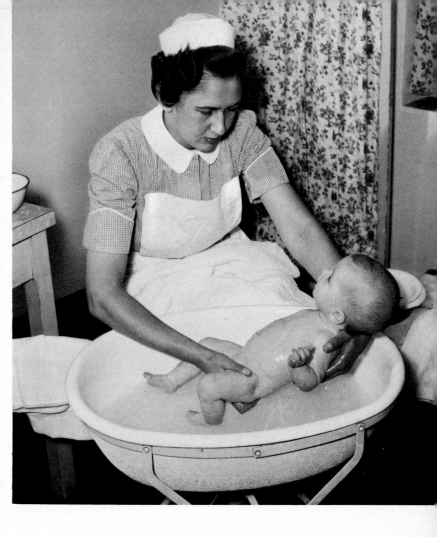

BATHING THE BABY

We are grateful to Camera Talks Limited for permission to reproduce this illustration from their colour filmstrip *Bathing Your Baby*.

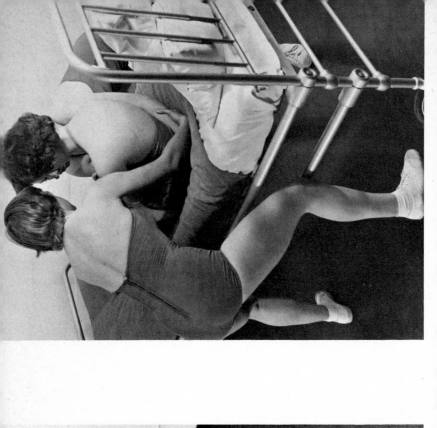

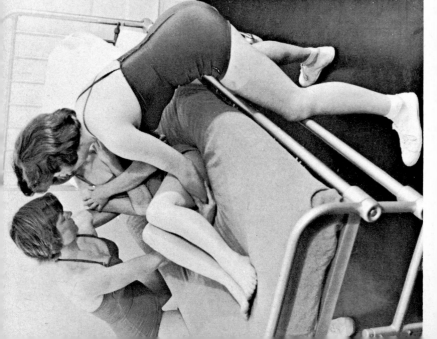

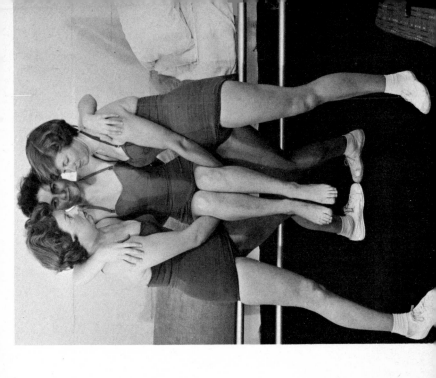

ORTHODOX LIFT

The illustrations above show the first of two methods of lifting a patient up the bed—the orthodox lift. Note the position of the lifters' hands under the patient's thighs in the left-hand photograph above. The right-hand photograph above is the rear view showing the position of the lifters' feet and legs and the posture of the head and back. Note the position of the lifters' hands in relation to the patient's sacrum. The patient is moved by the lifters straightening their legs and transferring their weight in the direction of the movement.

The photograph on the right shows the patient being lifted from the bed to a chair. Note particularly the bended knees of the lifters, and the position of their feet. The lifters' hands support the small of the patient's back.

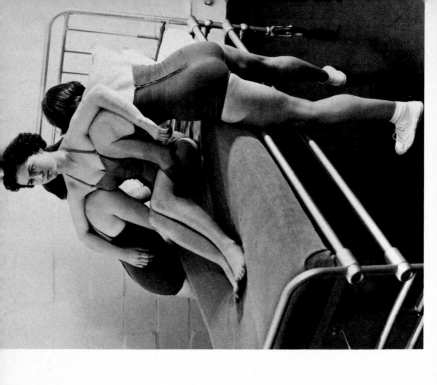
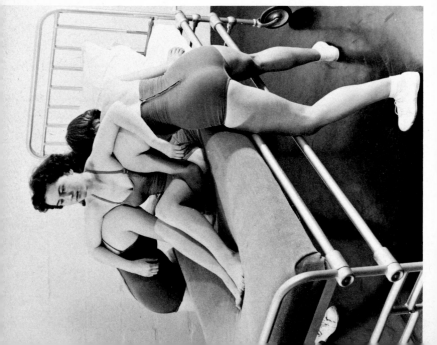

SHOULDER LIFT 1

The two photographs above illustrate the second method of lifting the patient up the bed. The left-hand illustration shows the starting position. Note the general position of the lifters in relation to the patient. It is essential that the lifters stand level with the patient's hips. One lifter grasps the other's forearm under the patient's thighs, and each presses her shoulder into the patient's axilla. The patient should be asked to rest her arms lightly on the lifters' backs. The right-hand illustration shows the lift. Having pressed her shoulder into the patient's axilla, each lifter smoothly extends her hips and knees and transfers her weight onto the forward leg. Throughout the movement the lifters stand as close to the bed as possible. Note that the shoulder lift cannot be used if the patient has injuries to the upper part of the trunk, shoulder or arms.

With the two types of shoulder lift shown above and on the following pages there is the disadvantage that the nurses cannot watch the patient's face for signs of pain or other discomfort, therefore they should be sure to ask the patient to tell them if she is uncomfortable in any way.

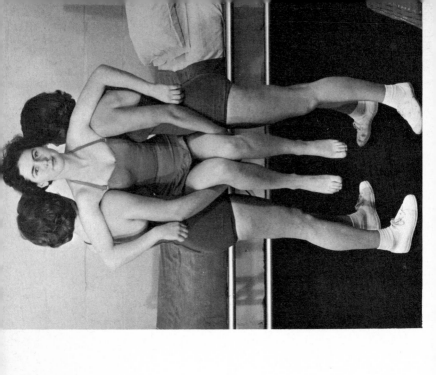
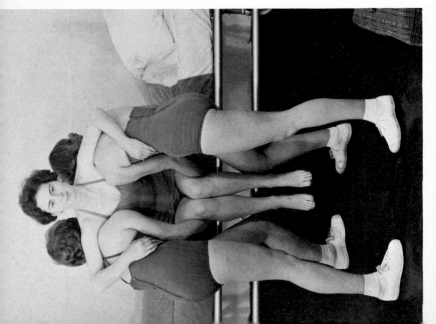

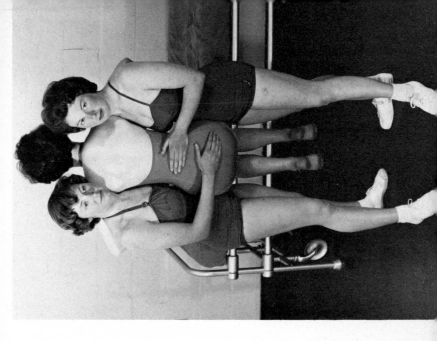

SHOULDER LIFT II

This method can also be used to lift the patient from the bed to a chair. The left-hand photograph shows the starting position. The lift is illustrated in the right-hand photograph above. Having lifted the patient from the bed, each lifter's free hand is placed so as to support the small of the patient's back. When necessary one lifter can use this free hand to carry an object such as a tube or an infusion bottle. After lifting, the lifters turn in an agreed direction to face the chair.

The illustrations of the Orthodox Lift and the two Shoulder Lifts are reproduced by kind permission of the Chartered Society of Physiotherapy from their publication *Lifting Patients in Hospital*.

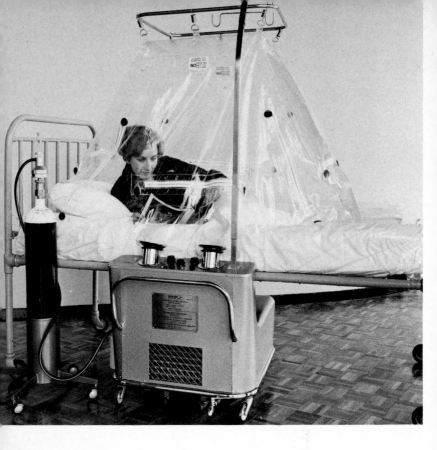

OXYGEN TENT

In this refrigerated tent oxygen concentrations, humidity and temperature are easily controllable. Visibility is good through the canopy which also allows plenty of room for movement. This patient should perhaps have been given another pillow.

We wish to thank Vickers Limited for permission to use the above photograph.

Preparations for Performing Simple Surgical Dressings

All the work done in the operating theatre and on the surgical ward aims at the prevention of sepsis, so preparations for performing dressings should be made with fastidious care and before commencing to lay her trolley and again before doing any dressing or touching any object which has been rendered sterile, the nurse must get her hands as clean as it is possible to make them.

With experience the enrolled nurse will learn how to avoid touching any article which is not sterile after she has washed her hands, and by using sterile forceps to use the non-touch technique whenever dealing with a wound, however small. She will cover her nose and mouth with a disposable mask so that she cannot infect the patient with bacteria in her own droplet spray (see p. 138).

PREPARING THE DRESSING TROLLEY

The trolley is swabbed over with antiseptic and dried with a paper towel.

Top shelf:

Covered sterile bowl containing dressings and towels
Covered sterile instrument tray containing four pairs of dissecting forceps
Covered sterile bowl containing gallipots
Tall jar containing Cheatle's forceps in disinfectant

Bottom shelf:

Lotions e.g. Cetavlon, eusol, ether
Tray containing bandages, strapping, scissors, safety pins. Disposal bags clipped to the sides of the trolley, or jar of disinfectant for dirty instruments and closed bin for dirty dressings

F

METHOD OF PERFORMING A SIMPLE DRESSING

Arrange the bedclothes so that the patient is uncovered as little as possible.

Remove the bandages and outer dressing and discard them.

Wash your hands thoroughly and dry them on a paper towel.

Using forceps, remove the wound dressing. If it has stuck swab it gently with sterile normal saline or sterile water until it comes away easily. Never pull it off.

Place dressing and forceps in the disposal bags, or in the containers.

Using fresh forceps place sterile towels round the wound.

Clean around the wound, always swabbing away from the wound, not towards it. Use each swab once only.

Cover the wound with a fresh dressing, then discard the forceps into the bag or container.

Apply a fresh bandage and see that the dressing is held firmly and comfortably.

Re-arrange the bedclothes.

Clean the trolley and set it afresh before going on to the next patient.

Sterile packs

If your hospital has a CSSD you will be working with packs which will probably contain towels, dressings, swabs, gallipots and dissecting forceps.

When the outer wrapper is removed the pack can be placed on the top of the trolley and the inner wrapper opened out to provide a sterile towel on which the dressings, gallipots and instruments can be arranged.

Additional equipment such as forceps for arranging the contents of the pack, scissors, clip removers, or drainage tubing, will be sterilized in individual packs, and used as required.

SWABBING AND CLEANSING THE VULVA

This treatment is carried out for a few days after most operations on the female genital tract, i.e. gynaecological operations.

Required:

Top shelf

Covered sterile bowl containing swabs, vulval pads, gauze dressings

Covered sterile tray containing two pairs dissecting forceps

Covered sterile bowl of lotion for swabbing, e.g. normal saline, plain water, or antiseptic as ordered

Bottom shelf

Clean T bandage

Disposal bags clipped to trolley sides, or jar of disinfectant for dirty forceps and covered container for dirty dressings

Method. Turn back the bedclothes and arrange a small blanket over the patient's chest and abdomen.

Wash your hands.

Turn the lower bedclothes back with your elbow.

Separate the labia with your left hand and hold them apart while you gently swab the vulva with your right hand.

Start at the outer aspect of the vulva and work inwards.

Swab from above downwards.

Use each swab once only.

Place the clean vulval pad in position.

Ask the patient to close her thighs and turn on her left side.

Turn back the pad to expose the perineum.

Using forceps dry the stitch area with a sterile swab and apply a fresh dressing.

Discard the forceps.

Cover the dressing with the pad and fix it in place with a T bandage.

Arrange the bedclothes over the patient and leave her comfortable.

Jug douche

If a jug douche is ordered you will need, in addition to the articles above:

Top shelf

Sterile 2 pint jug of warm lotion, e.g. normal saline, plain
 water, or antiseptic as ordered, at 38° C (100° F)
Lotion thermometer

Bottom shelf

Plastic square to protect the bottom sheet
Bedpan and cover

Method. After swabbing the vulva place the patient on the bedpan.

Part the labia and pour the lotion over the vulva.

Dry carefully with sterile swabs.

Remove the bedpan.

Apply a vulval pad and continue with dressing the stitch area.

17

Diseases Affecting all Systems of the Body

There are certain serious diseases which are commonly met with but which we could not discuss under any particular system, because they are able, either immediately or later on, to affect any part of the body.

Cancer

This is a vast subject which can be dealt with only very briefly here—whole books have been written on cancer of one organ alone.

You will often hear the word 'tumour' or 'growth'.

The cells which normally go to form a tissue or organ grow in an orderly, planned fashion, and when that organ has reached its proper size, growth stops, except for occasional repair operations. In the case of a tumour, however, these cells, for no apparent reason, just go on multiplying or increasing until there are so many of them that a lump appears, or, if deep down in the body, it starts pressing on nerves or other structures nearby and so causing discomfort of some kind.

There are two kinds of these 'new growths', one of which happily is harmless. They are:

1. *Benign or innocent tumours*

These are quite common, and do no great harm as they 'keep

155

themselves to themselves', as it were. They grow neatly in one place, often inside a capsule, and do not spread.

They are easy to remove, and as a rule do not occur again.

Examples: *(a)* Papilloma, which grows out from the skin, such as a wart.

(b) Adenoma, which grows in glands, often in the neck.

(c) Lipoma, made from fat; it may occur anywhere.

(d) Myoma, made from muscle cells. The commonest ones of all are the fibroids that so many women have removed from the uterus.

So the first thing to realize is that a tumour does not always mean cancer.

The second thing that everybody should know is that if there is any reason to suspect that a growth *has* started somewhere, the sooner they get medical advice the more chance there is of a permanent cure, even if it does turn out to be cancerous.

Unfortunately the word cancer has come to hold so much fear for the average person that many are afraid to go to the doctor lest they should be told they have got the thing they dread, whereas if they went at once they might well be spared months of anxiety by learning that it is, perhaps, only a lipoma after all; while if it is indeed cancer they may save their lives by having early treatment.

2. *Malignant tumours—Cancer*

These tumours are so-called because cancer means a crab, and these cells seem to send out claws in all directions. These growths do not stop at a certain point like the benign ones, but keep growing and what is worse, cells also get broken off and carried by the lymph and blood stream into other parts of the body, to start up new 'secondary' growths.

There are two types:

(a) Carcinoma. This is by far the commonest type. These growths can occur on the skin (rodent ulcers), in the breast, the

uterus, bladder, stomach, intestine, lungs, and even in the mouth and throat.

(b) Sarcoma. This occurs in connective tissue, such as bone, and tends to affect the very young or the old rather than those of middle years.

The symptoms will, of course, vary according to the organ first affected, but certain things should always be investigated:

1. Any abnormal bleeding or discharge.
2. Persistent loss of weight that is not the result of dieting.
3. Any lump in, or change in the appearance of the breasts.
4. Any continuous discomfort, like indigestion, cough, hoarseness, not relieved by ordinary means.
5. One thing you will notice missing—pain. THERE WILL BE NO PAIN in the early stages. This absence of pain, Nature's warning signal in most diseases, is what makes cancer such a terrible problem. So many people think 'It can't be anything much because it does not hurt'. The pain will come—later—but by then it may be too late.

Treatment. This, according to the site, type and extent of the trouble, will include: surgery—complete removal of the affected area, if possible; radiation by either deep X-rays or Cobalt Bomb or the insertion of radium. These latter methods destroy the growing cells.

Afterwards, a regular check-up is performed, from month to month, to watch over the patient, so that relief is at hand if there is any further trouble.

Tuberculosis

This is one of the oldest diseases known to man. It existed thousands of years ago, in all countries, affecting both man and animals.

At last this grave infection is being conquered. But even if the nurse may not see many new cases, she may see people whom the disease crippled in youth, or who still carry its complications in some form.

There are three types:

1. *Pulmonary tuberculosis*

Tuberculosis of the lungs is the commonest because it is the most easily spread. The germ causing it, the tubercle bacillus, lives on human tissues and is not spread by animals. The disease develops very slowly, so there are not usually any dramatic symptoms to show what is happening. Thus the disease may have a good hold before it is recognized.

The early symptoms are generally a feeling of being tired and unwell (malaise). There is a cough with sputum, and sometimes a pain in the chest, while if the temperature was taken it would be found to be irregular, often up in the morning and normal at night. There is loss of appetite and of weight. In women the periods may stop. A characteristic and suspicious symptom is excessive sweating, especially in bed at night.

Sometimes the patient may cough up bright red, frothy blood—*haemoptysis*. Although this may be very frightening, it may be a good thing, as it will send the patient to the doctor, and investigations and treatment will be started at once.

Treatment. As soon as the X-rays, sputum examination and other tests reveal that tuberculosis is present, the patient is put to bed on complete rest. He may be sent to a sanatorium or chest hospital, where he will be properly looked after, and where he will not be able to infect his family.

A good, rich, appetizing diet is given, with added vitamins. Modern treatment by drugs has cured many who once would have died. These are *streptomycin, para-aminosalicylic acid* (PAS), and *isoniazid* (INAH).

In some cases surgery helps, either by putting the diseased lung out of action so that it can rest completely (artificial pneumothorax) or even by removing parts of the lung altogether (lobectomy). The whole treatment may take many months, but most patients are cured and able to go back to lead a normal life.

Prevention. This is a disease that can be prevented. Better living conditions and proper food have made people healthier and less liable to catch it. Mass X-ray units that travel round to every town and village find many early cases which can be treated quickly.

The Mantoux Test is a skin test done to see if individuals are liable to get tuberculosis. If they are, a vaccine called BCG is available for anyone exposed to infection—people like nurses or medical students.

2. *Bovine tuberculosis*

This condition is caused by drinking milk from infected cows. Instead of affecting the lungs it gets into bones, joints, the peritoneum or the glands in the neck. It has been responsible for much crippling of young children, who often had to spend years in an orthopaedic hospital.

Prevention of this crippling disease has been carried out by the better care of cows and their milk. All cows are now Tuberculin Tested and protected from tuberculosis, while all milk is pasteurized. Thus the bovine type is practically stamped out in all countries with a modern health and hygiene service.

3. *Miliary tuberculosis*

This occurs when, instead of settling in the lungs only, the germs are spread in the blood stream all over the body. It is from this type that tuberculous meningitis arises. It can occur in young children before they have got immunity against it. Fortunately it is a rare condition now and, when it does occur, the use of modern antibiotics saves most of these cases.

The Venereal Diseases

These are infections passed from one to another through sexual intercourse. Like tuberculosis, their history goes right back through the ages.

Unfortunately, we have not been able to get rid of them as we have almost conquered tuberculosis. The reason for this is that, although antibiotic drugs are available and will cure any case in its early stages, the cause and the shame attached to it by many of the victims make them afraid to go to a doctor, so they go untreated. They themselves have to endure the consequences of this neglect and, worse still, they may pass the disease on to somebody else. It is easy to understand this reluctance to seek advice, but it is quite unnecessary. The staff in venereal disease clinics understand how patients feel and treatment is completely confidential. Hospitals treating venereal disease are listed in most public lavatories and a letter from the patient's general practitioner is not required before making an appointment. There are two chief venereal diseases.

1. *Syphilis*

This is caused by a germ called a spirochaete, which usually gets into the body through the mucous membrane of the genito-urinary tract. It is a very serious disease which can not only affect any organ or tissue, but even after it seems to have subsided, wakes up again many years after the victim has forgotten the early symptoms. Worst of all, syphilis can be passed on from mother to child. There are three stages:

1. A primary sore, called a chancre, which becomes a deep ulcer, appears, usually somewhere on the genital organs.
2. Secondary symptoms appear a month or so later, the organism having multiplied and spread. Now the patient becomes ill with a sore throat, swollen glands, often a rash. White streaks may be seen in the throat—'snail-track' ulcers.
3. Tertiary or third-stage syphilis occurs long after the victim seems to have got better. The disease may now show itself by the destruction of a great blood vessel like the aorta, by weakening its walls and causing what is called an aneurysm —a patch that balloons out like a blister and may burst, causing a terrible haemorrhage and sudden death. In some people gumma or swellings occur in organs such as the liver or the brain. In others a form of insanity may appear, with destruction of normal mental powers, and

paralysis of the body as well. This is called General Paralysis of the Insane—you may hear it called GPI for short. Because people are seeking treatment earlier this stage is rarely seen now.

The only effective treatment is early diagnosis and medical treatment. This usually consists of massive doses of procaine penicillin, given over a long period.

2. *Gonorrhoea*

This infection is caused by quite a different organism, a very small germ called the gonococcus.

First of all it causes inflammation, pain and soreness in the urethra and external genital organs. There is a discharge of pus, and the glands around are swollen and painful. Many complications can follow in both sexes. These include spread to the internal genital organs, which can lead to sterility (the inability to have children). Sometimes the germs are carried in the blood to joints, tendons, eyes, or lungs, or brain, giving rise to arthritis, iritis, pneumonia, or meningitis.

The eyes of newborn babies can also be badly infected, and if not properly treated at once, this can lead to blindness.

Treatment. Again, this depends on early diagnosis and the injection of large doses of penicillin in one of its forms, or one of the sulphonamide drugs may be used.

People should be taught to seek medical advice at once if they have reason to fear that they may have caught one of these diseases. If a nurse is consulted she can assure the sufferer that such advice and treatment will be given in strict confidence and secrecy.

18

Caring for Elderly Patients

The enrolled nurse often has to deal with elderly patients, and hers is a very special responsibility. Most of the old people who come into our hospitals for care and attention have lived good and useful lives, have reared families and sent them out into the world, have fought for their country, or in other ways have given of their best for many years. We must not let them feel helpless, passed over, forgotten, with existence becoming a misery as they lose their faculties and strength.

The changes that take place in old age are the common lot of us all. They include impairment of memory for recent events, the tendency to live in the past and to recount the same story over and over again, self-centredness and a dulling of the emotions, apparent greed and a desire for sweet things, and the demanding of personal attention. We must remember that the mental breakdown is brought about by the increasing handicap of an ageing body, and the burden of an accumulation of minor ailments, the slowing of the circulation, the hardening of the arteries and the degeneration of the brain cells. To be angry with the foibles of the aged is as foolish as to be angry with a year old baby for not showing the wisdom of an adult.

Wonderful things are being done today for old people by physical medicine. The bedridden are taught to walk again, the crippled to do for themselves many things that were impossible a few years ago. Nobody is too old today for successful treatment, but the most valued ally that geriatric medicine has is a team of workers who really understand their old patients, who treat them with dignity and respect, and who give them a sense of security and, above all, of being wanted. There is so much they can pass on to younger people from the wisdom which comes from experience. And if they do not always seem to be wise, but sometimes rather silly, obstinate or 'difficult', remember that age brings physical changes to the brain as well as other tissues. They must be encouraged hourly, never bullied or scolded, to make those movements or perform those tasks that are going to make them still useful members of the community for perhaps several years longer.

Perhaps the greatest reward that the nurse can have is to see a patient who has been bedridden for five years totter down the ward for the first time, or to see the arthritic hands making their first basket. There is more scope for nursing skill in geriatric nursing than in any other branch, and it needs the best of nurses.

The kinds of illnesses which affect the older patients are those which come through the ageing of their bodies, and the changes which take place in their tissues, rather than the short acute conditions of younger people, which are more often due to infection.

The branch of medicine and nursing which deals with the care of the aged is called Geriatrics.

A chronic disease means that, though often mild in nature, it is slow in its course and continues for a long time, perhaps for years. Here are some of them:

1. Heart disease, ending in congestive heart failure
2. Cancer
3. Cerebral haemorrhage with resulting hemiplegia (a stroke)
4. Arthritis
5. Parkinson's disease
6. Chronic bronchitis
7. Fractures, especially of the neck of the femur

8. Senility, with mental changes and general bodily neglect and undernourishment
9. Multiple or disseminated sclerosis

There are others, of course, but these are among the commonest in our hospital wards.

The complications which good nursing aims to prevent are:

1. *Pressure sores,* due to lying too long in one position, or to incontinence.
2. *Retention of the urine* and infection of the bladder.
3. *Constipation* which may lead to a serious condition called *volvulus,* which would require surgery.
4. *Contractures,* or unnatural formation of the limbs, due to leaving them too long in one position without exercise.
5. *Malnutrition,* because the patient may have very little appetite, or be 'faddy' about the food offered her.
6. *Pneumonia,* caused by poor circulation and saliva or particles of food passing down the trachea.
7. *Depression,* often due to loneliness, or to failing sight or hearing.

Ideally old people should have the support of a loving family around them, but unfortunately this is not always so.

Many old people live by themselves, perhaps in one room. There may be a flight of stairs to climb, and no lift. So they go out as little as possible. Cooking is a burden, so they live on bread and jam, biscuits, tinned stuff and cups of tea. They are not taking enough protein, vitamins and minerals, so they feel tired and unwell.

Perhaps no one visits them and they get depressed and apathetic. Why bother to have a bath or wash one's clothes? What does it matter? No one will notice anyway. When they do finally fall ill and are admitted to hospital the nurse may have the unpleasant task of cleaning up a dirty, truculent, possibly verminous old person.

As you go about this task try to remember that what you are seeing is not the real person. He is hidden somewhere underneath this cloak of physical illness, neglect and depression. The art of geriatric nursing lies in having the imagination and the skill to bring the real person to life again. The skill to nurse the physical illness, and the mental outlook as well.

This applies to all nursing, of course, but the need for it is seen very clearly in geriatric patients and you should try to keep these two aspects of your work in mind all the time.

Mealtimes

Nourishing food, taken regularly, will often bring about a surprising improvement in an old person's condition.

Remember that what he needs most is protein, vitamins and minerals, so get as much milk, eggs and fish into him as you can, and as he improves add meat, cheese, fruit and vegetables.

Make sure that patients who have dentures use them. If they keep taking them out there is probably something wrong with them. Let sister know so that they can be attended to.

Meals should be served punctually and as daintily and appetizingly as possible. *Hot* food must be served *hot* and *cold* food *cold*.

Make the tray as attractive as possible and arrange everything within easy reach of the patient. Crockery, cutlery and linen should be spotlessly clean. It is much better to use a plastic traycloth, which can be wiped clean, than a dirty linen one which cannot be changed because the clean laundry has not arrived.

Serve small portions and do not fill cups and glasses too full.

Vary the diet as much as possible, always obeying the doctor's orders.

Whenever possible sit the patient well up, see that his back is comfortably supported, and cover his shoulders with a bed jacket.

Pay special attention to the mouth and teeth, before and after meals, especially if the patient is taking a milk diet. Give water freely if allowed.

When feeding a helpless patient place a diet cloth under his chin and raise his head by placing your left arm under his pillow. Take plenty of time so that he does not feel hurried, and give small mouthfuls.

Clear away immediately the meal is over and do not leave unfinished drinks at the bedside.

Attend to the comfort of the patients both before and after meals, refilling hot water bottles, giving bedpans and urinals, and sponging hands and face. No painful dressing or treatment should be done near meal times.

Patients who can do so should get up and sit at a table in the ward.

See that they are seated on chairs of the right height so that they can reach their food without strain. If the chair is too low and you cannot change it, raise the patient on a cushion.

Arthritic patients are often helped by having handle bar grips on their cutlery. Any device which will enable a patient to feed himself is worth trying out, not only for the patient's sake but because in an overcrowded, understaffed geriatric ward it means that more nursing time can be given to the really helpless patients.

Remember with all patients that old people's taste buds are not as keen as those of younger people and they appreciate well seasoned food. Some, of course, will be on special diets, but for those who are not restricted the addition of salt and pepper, pickle, sauces or sugar in generous quantities may make all the difference between a meal well taken and one pushed aside.

Bowels

Old people and people suffering from chronic illness do not tolerate strong purgatives, but often require enemas. The disposable enemas are particularly useful here. Instead of a bedpan they should have a commode provided whenever they can use one, or be wheeled to the toilet.

It is worth finding out whether the patient has been in the

habit of taking a laxative regularly and what particular brand he has been using. When a habit has been established over a number of years it is not always wise to break it off completely, but much can be done to relieve constipation by including fruit and vegetables in the diet, in purée form if necessary, and by getting the patient moving. Even if he is unable to get up encourage him to move his legs up and down and to change his position frequently.

All pat[ients] ... as possible, partly because it will p... muscle wastage, but also because i... in bed they soon lose the will and ... health, both physical and mental, d...

If a pa... ay be possible to nurse him, for ... his feet on a footstool. This will ... re fully and relieve his distressed ... ypes of machines called hoists in u... can lift quite heavy people out ... eel- or arm-chair.

Old peop... nges in temperature and quickly ... they tend to move slowly and w... armly and comfortably clad, the... and their stockings changed frequ... see that they have clean handkerc... recious possessions like spectacles ... n to a Day Room or the Occupati... t to be able to lay their hands on ... cause them great distress.

Old people de[pend] ... on their feet. See that corns, ingrowing toe nails, bunions, and any other disability which makes walking difficult is reported at once, so that the chiropodist can attend to it.

Avoid slippers as much as you can. They give no support

167

to the feet and may cause old people to trip. Get them to wear their shoes and see that they are in good repair.

If old people need help when walking they should be supplied with walking sticks tipped with rubber, or a walking frame may be useful.

Floors in a geriatric ward should never be polished. A non-slip plastic finish is generally used. Rugs are dangerous and carpets should be inspected frequently for worn or threadbare patches which could cause an accident. Even a slight tumble can mean a broken leg for an old person because his bones are so brittle.

Occupation and Recreation

Stagnation of any kind leads to decay and unless old people live as regular and normal a life as possible and are provided with stimulating contacts, they deteriorate rapidly both physically and mentally.

They should have visitors, newspapers, books and magazines, and interesting hobbies, and should not be encouraged to regard themselves as chronic invalids. They should be placed under the care of the occupational therapist as soon as they are well enough.

Apart from physical care old people have two great needs. They need companionship and they need to feel that they still count as an individual person. Loneliness and the feeling that no one would really care if they died tomorrow are often the basic factors, which lead to depression, apathy, malnutrition and finally physical illness.

The nurse can do much to revive an old person's interest in life, and his self-esteem.

Look for any little way in which you can emphasise his individuality. If there is room in the ward for patients to have photos, or small personal belongings on their lockers, let them do so and make a point of talking about them whenever you can. No matter that he has already told you who the people in the photo are. Ask him again another day. Old people forget, and he won't wonder why you are asking again. Comment on any little article, a tobacco pouch, a sponge bag, a purse, 'Look Mr Brown, this is Mr White's wallet. His grandson made it for him at school, isn't it beautifully finished? Let's see Mr White, how old is he now?' and so on.

Keep a list of all the birthdays in the ward and make a little celebration of each one. It may be only birthday wishes and telling the others, but perhaps the kitchen can provide a birthday cake as well. This is often possible if they are given enough warning.

Don't be put off if a cake is out of the question. It is the remembering that counts most. Try to keep a little extra jam in store, or an extra packet of biscuits, just to mark the occasion, or put out a packet of brightly coloured paper serviettes. And don't stop at birthdays, be on the lookout for any little happening which will give you an excuse to draw attention to a patient, as an individual person. 'Mrs Green walked the full length of the ward today. It's the first time she has managed it—let's have a singsong this evening to celebrate!' 'Mr Black's son has just been promoted works manager, we've only got tea but all the same we'll drink his health.' If you make a habit of thinking in this way you will soon have plenty of ideas.

Patients who can get up can play cards, Ludo, draughts, or watch television. Some of those in bed may be able to make baskets, do some knitting or crochet, or read the newspaper.

Others may be too frail or too disabled to do any of these things. More than anything else they need someone to talk with them. This can be difficult for a nurse in a busy ward, but try to remember, every time you give them nursing care, to exchange a few words with them as well. The important thing is that it should be an *exchange*. So many nurses chatter at patients thinking they are cheering them up, but the flow of talk goes over the old person's head. He is bemused and cannot take it in, so he makes no response.

Not all old people are deaf, so don't shout unless it is absolutely necessary. Keep your voice at the normal level, but get the old person's attention before you start. Say his name, or touch him, and wait until he is looking directly at you before you go on. When you have said something to him, wait for him to answer you. It may be thirty seconds or more before he can get the words out, but go on with what you are doing and give him time. Two sentences spoken by the patient to you is worth more than any amount of bright talk on your part if he cannot respond.

Visitors

Visitors can be the life blood of a geriatric ward. They keep the patient in touch with the outside world, with home and the family, with friends and neighbours.

Do all that you possibly can to let visitors know that they are welcome. Tell them how pleased the nursing staff are to see them. Try to learn their names, and use them. If you see a visitor struggling to make conversation with a patient but having no success, go along and help. Sometimes visitors feel they can be of some use by feeding the patient. Make a point of going out of your way to thank them for it.

In between visits try to get patients to write to their visitors. If they cannot do so themselves, offer to write for them. A short, simple note is all that is necessary, just to say how much the patient enjoyed the visit and that he is looking forward to seeing the visitor again. Visitors should be your valued partners in the effort to rehabilitate the patient.

Spiritual Care

Spiritual comfort may be a great help to old people, and the nurse must see that such help is available from the patient's church or the visiting clergyman. It should be possible to have the bible read to those who cannot read themselves, and for them to hear broadcast services in the wards. They enjoy the community singing of hymns and a nurse who can play the piano can bring them much pleasure.

Sleep

All the skill of the night nurse may be needed to help elderly people through the night (p. 89).

Sedatives should be used as sparingly as possible because the effect tends to carry over into the day. A patient who is restless during the night is given a sedative. He settles and sleeps, but in the morning he is still partly under the influence of the drug. He doesn't want to wake up, dozes off again over his breakfast, is apathetic when the occupational therapist comes round, sleeps most of the morning, doesn't want to get up or to talk, and may be rather muddled in his thinking. He is not really alert again until the late afternoon. When bedtime comes he naturally doesn't feel like going to sleep and is wakeful and restless after lights out, so another sedative is given and a vicious circle is set up.

The good practical nurse uses all her nursing skill to get the patient to sleep without drugs whenever possible. Fortunately old people generally wake early in the normal course of events, and like an early start to the day, so that the morning activities can proceed in an unhurried atmosphere. One of the best preparations for a good night's sleep is a day which is as active and enjoyable as the patient's condition will permit, and this is how you should approach the problem with old people.

Care of the Dying

The essential qualities of nursing are best seen in the attitude of a nurse to the dying. Her kindly care of the patient and sympathetic consideration towards his relatives may do much to lighten his passing and comfort those who are left.

She will do her best to bring to the bedside in good time the clergyman and any other person whom the patient would like to see.

She will attend to his comfort by:

1. Keeping him warm

2. Changing his position occasionally
3. Seeing that his head rests comfortably on the pillow
4. Keeping his mouth clean and moist
5. Bathing his eyes if there is any discharge
6. Staying with him if he is alone, or within call if his friends are by his side
7. Touching his hand gently from time to time, even if he appears to be unconscious, to let him know that she is with him

Death brings sadness not only to the patient's relatives, but to the nurses and the other patients as well.

If you have not yet seen anyone die it may help you to know that most people lose consciousness for several hours beforehand. Although the patient's breathing may be difficult he is unaware of pain.

Many patients fear that their pain will increase as death approaches, but in fact the reverse is true, and they and their relatives should have the comfort of being told this. Pain is nearly always less during the hours before death and often seems to leave the patient entirely, even if he is conscious.

The realization that death is coming seems to dawn gradually, whether he has been told of its approach or not. Many, especially the old and those who have had a long illness, relax as death draws near, as if glad to be leaving their weariness behind. Death itself comes peacefully and almost imperceptibly.

Grief is a healing emotion. A mature nurse understands this and will not make anxious efforts to stop relatives' tears, although she will do all she can to comfort them. Often the best comfort is someone who will stay quietly beside them until the first anguish has passed, and will give them the assurance that everything possible was done for the patient.

As you become senior try to remember that the younger, or more junior nurses may be deeply disturbed by a patient's death. They may be appalled at the sudden death of a young person, realizing, perhaps for the first time, that this could happen to them. They may feel disgust and relief at the death of a patient with, for example, cancer of the face, and may hate themselves for feeling like this. Or they may experience a real loss and personal sorrow after the death of someone towards whom they had come to feel affection and admiration.

The needs of grieving relatives for comfort and reassurance, and the nursing care which must continue to be given to the other patients in the ward, often prevent nurses from expressing their feelings at the time, but later, when the rush of work has slackened, it helps to sit down together with a cup of tea and just share the experience.

Poor Mr A. has gone at last, and all little Nurse B. can feel is a deep thankfulness that she will never have to do his dressings again. She feels guilty and ashamed about it, and worries over it when she goes off duty. It will make all the difference to her attitude, both to her work and to herself, if she can become aware that other nurses feel like this too. She may then be able to accept her feelings, instead of trying to deny them, and so draw from the experience a deeper understanding of human nature.

Nurse C. tries desperately not to let anyone see that she has been crying in the sluice because dear Mrs G has died. Becoming fond of a patient is not a crime, and it is the most natural thing in the world to grieve when he or she dies. The more we can understand and accept our own feelings the more likely we are to be able to help other people, whether they are patients or staff, and a good way to start understanding is to talk about it together.

Last Offices

After the end has come, take the relatives outside and give them tea. Make sure that they see the sister or a doctor, and that they know where to go for any necessary certificates. Then return to the ward and strip the bed of inessentials such as appliances or pillows. Remove all top bedclothes except a sheet. Remove the personal clothing and lay the body flat with the limbs straight. Close the eyes by placing small pads of damp cotton wool over them. If there were dentures, these should be replaced now and a bandage tied round the jaw to keep it closed. An hour later prepare what is required for performing the last offices.

Articles needed for performing the last offices

Bowl of warm water, soap and flannels, non-absorbent wool for plugging orifices, sinus forceps, dressing forceps, scissors, nail scissors, brush and comb, receivers, tape.

Antiseptic, lint, jaconet, bandage, needle and thread.

Gown, two large sheets, labels with patient's name, age, date, time of death, ward.

Method. The body should be washed and dried thoroughly. Anus and vagina are plugged with grey wool. If there is a wound, any tubes must be removed and clean dressing applied and strapped on.

A clean gown or shroud is put on. The nails should be cleaned and trimmed, and the hair combed and arranged becomingly. The hands may be crossed on the breast. The eyes should be closed reverently. It may be necessary to keep the jaw closed with a bandage for an hour or two until rigor mortis sets in. One label should be tied round wrist or ankle.

Clean sheets are then put on the bed, one covering the body completely until it is time for removal to the mortuary. The second label is attached to the top sheet.

The porter responsible should be informed when you are ready, and arrangements will be made to remove the body to the mortuary. Afterwards, all linen will be sent to the laundry, the mattress and pillows to be disinfected in some way suitable to the material of which they are made, the bedstead and locker washed, and disinfected. The bed is then made up with clean bedding, the floor swept, the screens removed, and everything should look bright and clean so that any unhappy impression there may be will soon fade from the minds of the other patients.

Disposal of the patient's property after death

When a patient dies in hospital, unless the relatives have given instructions to the contrary, all jewellery should be removed and handed, with other possessions, to the ward sister, who has the responsibility of returning them to the nearest relative.

19

Looking After Children

THE NORMAL INFANT

The normal infant at birth is plump, with well-rounded limbs, short, fat neck and full cheeks. The skin is a brighter red over the soles of the feet and the palms of the hands than elsewhere and there are red blotches about the face due to the fact that the blood of a young infant contains more red cells than that of an older child or an adult. These red blotches must not be confused with rashes and bruises, which the nurse must report at once to the doctor.

The weight is about 7 lb. at birth, but owing to improved ante-natal care the weight is tending to increase. As a rule, the baby loses a few ounces of its birth weight during the first three days but regains it by the tenth day.

The child should gain about 6 ounces per week in the first three months, after which it progresses at a slightly lower rate. The normal weight for a child of one year is about 21 lb., and for a child of six years about 45 lb.

The child should have all its first teeth by the age of 2½ years. Eruption of the second teeth starts at about 6 years of age, and by the twelfth year all except the wisdom teeth are present.

About the end of the fourth month the baby will be able to distinguish objects with its eyes. It will be disturbed by loud or sudden noises, although more gentle sounds are only gradually appreciated.

A baby should begin to lift up its head by the fourth month.

At six months it should sit comfortably.

At ten months it should stand with support.

At twelve months it should begin to talk and from twelve to eighteen months it should begin to walk.

Sleep is a very important factor in mental and physical development. The baby must be placed comfortably in its cot, and the nurse must see that there is plenty of cool fresh air without draughts and that the covering is light and warm. If the child is left in the open air, care must be taken to protect its eyes from the sun.

An infant should sleep whenever it is not being fed, bathed, or having exercise. Until it is 4 years of age, a child needs an afternoon sleep daily.

Exercise. The older baby needs exercise so that its muscles and limbs may develop properly. It should be placed on a blanket in the play-pen or other safe place and allowed to kick freely for about half an hour before a feed is due at least twice a day.

Fresh air is essential as exposure to the light and ultra-violet rays produce vitamin D under the baby's skin.

Identity tapes are worn round the wrist or ankle and the nurse must report at once when they have become tight and need renewing.

Clothing

Clothes should be suitable for the season. They should be light in weight, warm and absorbent. Overclothing causes rashes, sweating, dehydration and then constipation.

Care must be taken to shield its head and particularly its ears from draughts.

Bathing

At first a baby is bathed once a day, in the morning, then later on when it is more active it is usually bathed morning and evening.

The room must be warm and free from draughts.

Everything likely to be needed must be placed in readiness and the clothes put to warm.

The temperature of the water should be about 40° C (100° F). It must always be tested with a bath thermometer and stirred with the hand, and the cold water must be placed in the bath before the hot.

Prepare:
> Two soft towels
> Superfatted soap
> Petroleum jelly
> Disposable napkins
> Safety pins, which must *always* be closed

Tray for swabbing eyes containing:
> Sterile boracic lotion
> Sterile swabs
> Receiver for used swabs

Method:

The nurse should wear a mackintosh apron and should tuck a towel round her waist.

She should then wash her hands and:

1. Swab the baby's eyes, using each swab once only, swabbing from the inner to the outer corner of the eye.
2. Swab and dry the face, but without using soap.
3. Wash and dry the hair, holding the baby under the left arm over the bath.
4. With the baby on her knee, lather its body with soap, then placing the left arm under the child's head and back and holding its legs with the right hand, lower it gently into the bath.
5. After splashing it with water to remove the soap and stimulate the skin, wrap it in a towel and pat it dry.
6. Apply petroleum jelly to the creases of the skin and buttocks.

7. If the stump of the umbilical cord has not separated, apply powder, a dressing, and a crepe bandage, using a large blanket stitch which can easily be cut off.
8. Put on the vest and napkins.
9. Draw the clothes on over the feet.

Remove soiled linen at once, and remember that warmth, fresh air, cleanliness and dryness are essential.

The baby should wear a warm nightgown but must not be overloaded with bedclothes.

Feeding

Human milk is best adapted to the needs of the normal infant. It is the right temperature, contains no germs, and possesses special substances which protect the infant from infection. Breast feeding is ideal because of these things, and because it brings mother and child into close contact, so giving the baby that sense of security and love that is his greatest need.

The nurse should make sure that the nipple is in the baby's mouth and that the child is swallowing the feed.

When human milk is insufficient or unobtainable, humanized cow's milk is given instead.

Proprietary preparations as a rule are too expensive for use in the average home but, when necessary, National Dried Milk may be obtained at a low price from Clinics or Welfare Centres, and is ideal because besides containing all the necessary ingredients for a proper diet, it is sterile.

An example of a feed for a 12 lb. infant:

Full cream dried milk	5 measures
Sugar	$1\frac{1}{2}$ teaspoons
Water	6 oz.

Babies are fed either 3- or 4-hourly up to the age of 9 months, and it can safely be assumed that the quantity is correct when the child increases normally in weight, does not vomit, and has healthy stools.

Some people like babies to be fed 'on demand', i.e. when they cry and appear to be hungry.

Before preparing any feed a nurse must put on a mask and wash her hands. Everything she uses must be sterilized. All the ingredients must be measured.

During feeding, the child is held in the nurse's arms with his head and back supported. The feed should be given slowly, taking about 10 to 20 minutes, and the teat is kept full so that air will not be swallowed.

The baby should be held up against the nurse's shoulder halfway through the feed, so that any wind can be brought up.

The bottle should be kept warm by placing it in a jug of hot water and the contents of an unfinished bottle must be thrown away.

A baby needs to be loved, to be held close and cuddled. Caressing and playing with a baby is a vital part of his nursing care, and the nurse should always find time for this after each feed. No baby should ever have to take his feed alone, with the bottle propped up beside him.

Babies' bottles should be rinsed in cold water after use and washed thoroughly in warm, soapy water, using a bottle brush. They should be left sterilized in a solution of Milton 1:80.

Teats must be rubbed with salt to remove the slime from the milk, turned and rinsed well, boiled for 2 minutes, and then stored in a covered jar.

Bottles and teats should be boiled once a day to keep them clean, and always if there has been any question of infection. Each baby should have its own bottle and teats and these must be labelled in order to avoid any baby being given those belonging to another one.

THE SICK CHILD

ADMISSION

When admitting a child you will need the usual information about his name, age, address, etc. (p. 66). In addition, if the patient is a baby ask the mother the type of feed he is having, how frequently he is fed, his weight and progress, whether vaccinated or immunized, if he has been christened and whether he has had any infectious disease or been in contact with one. If the baby is breast fed, special arrangements should be made for the mother to continue this at the hospital.

With toddlers and older children find out what the child calls his potty, or what he says when he wants to go to the lavatory. This is most important because some children are desperately shy. Hospital is no place for putting them through the anxiety of learning new ways. The sick child needs all the security he can get and one way of helping him is to use the words and phrases he has been taught at home.

Enquire about his bedtime routine. If you look back to your own childhood you will know the sort of things to ask. Is he afraid of the dark? Does he have a favourite object that he likes to take to bed? Is there a rhyme to be said, a goodnight phrase to be exchanged, or a prayer?

Let his mother stay as long as she can, and help with the routine of temperature taking, getting undressed, bathing, and going to bed. Introduce him to some of the other children while she is still there to give him confidence. Remember that a happy child makes a better recovery than one who is miserable. Anything you can do to lessen his fears is good nursing.

SETTLING DOWN

Make use of the information you have gained to help him begin to feel at home in the ward. Talk to him about his brothers and sisters, his hobbies, his schoolmates, the holidays, all the things which are familiar to him. Try to be a link between hospital and home, and remember to share your information with the other nurses so that they can help too.

Tell him about the other children in the ward. Most children will mix quite happily, but there will always be one or two who are quiet and hold back. These are the ones who specially need your care.

Tell him about the people who come and go in the ward—

the pathology laboratory technician, the school teacher, the occupational therapist, the dietitian. He will feel apprehensive of all staff at first, thinking that they are coming to do something horrible to him. But when you point out what fun the others are having with the teacher, and how clever John is in helping the man from the pathology laboratory he will not be quite so scared when his turn comes.

OBSERVATION

A child may contract practically the same diseases as an adult, but because of its more delicately balanced nervous system it reacts much more quickly to its environment and, in a very short time, trifling causes may produce grave symptoms.

On the other hand, a child may become exhausted and have a subnormal temperature but have apparently no symptoms of disease; it may then be very gravely ill. For this reason a nurse must be on the alert to notice any change in a child's condition, and must exercise great care in taking and charting the temperature, pulse and respiration.

Children are unable to stand a long period of starvation before operation, so the surgeon usually orders them to have glucose or barley sugar. After the operation is over, the nurse must take the child's temperature, pulse and respiration oftener and test the urine more frequently than is necessary in the case of an adult.

Bowel movements should be observed very carefully and if abnormal stools are observed the doctor should be informed. At first, an infant passes unformed, darkish green stools, then the colour becomes yellow and the stool the consistency of mustard. It does not become brown and formed until starch is included in the diet.

Frequent dark green small motions in an older baby are an indication that the baby is not having sufficient feeds, while large green motions prove, as do large bulky motions, that a baby is being over-fed.

Hard crumbly motions are a sign of constipation.

Pale motions may be a sign of serious disorder and should be reported to the doctor.

Fat in the stools may mean pancreatic disorder.

Curds in the stool prove that the feed is not being digested and needs diluting.

A grey, alkaline, offensive, crumbly stool is a proof that the feed contains too much protein, while an unformed, yellowish brown, frothy, acid stool proves that it contains too much sugar.

Slime or mucus in a stool indicates that there is inflammation or irritation of the bowel.

As in the case of an adult, pain will be reflected in the child's expression, e.g.:

Pain in the head will make a child contract his forehead.

Pain in the chest will cause sharpness of the nostrils.

Pain in the abdomen causes a drawing in of the upper lip.

Much can be learnt from the cry of a child

A normal cry is loud and strong and the child becomes red in the face.

A feeble wail or a fretful whine indicates pain and exhaustion.

A shrill piercing cry is often a symptom of brain disease.

A hoarse, throaty cry is a symptom of laryngitis.

Loud crying with movements of the arms and legs denotes hunger or a sudden attack of pain.

A paroxysmal piercing cry, relieved by the passage of flatus, is usually a symptom of indigestion.

TREATMENT

Never lie to a child. You need not go into the full truth in all its details, but it should never be necessary to tell him a lie. Once he finds that you didn't tell him the truth he will not trust you again. You have added to his anxiety, and to that extent you have delayed his recovery.

If the treatment is going to hurt you should tell him so.

Say something like, 'You'll feel a sharp prick, and then it will all be finished,' or 'It stings a bit, but it only lasts a minute', or 'It doesn't really *hurt*, but it feels a bit funny', so that he knows what to expect.

If he must be held while a procedure is carried out, do it firmly but kindly as well. Hold him close against you and soothe his fear by talking to him. If you can hold his hand at the same time as you restrain him, do so.

Don't think that if you suddenly descend on him without warning and pin his arms to his sides you will get the procedure over quickly and he will forget all about it. He won't. This is the way to build up fear and tension, to delay his recovery and perhaps to lay the foundations of a life-long dread of hospitals.

Explain simply and quietly what has to be done, and that it will help to make him better. The more he has learnt to trust you the more cooperation you will get.

VISITING

Children cannot be reasoned with like adults. The younger the child the harder it is for him to understand why his mother has to leave him just at the time when he needs her most of all. The bewilderment and unhappiness he goes through at this time may have a permanent effect on his emotional development.

It is now recognized that all children in hospital should be visited as frequently and for as long as possible, and that the mothers of children under five should be with their children all the time.

So important is the mother's presence that the Minister of Health has said that all hospitals should allow open visiting in children's wards.

Most hospitals are doing this, but some still insist on fixed visiting hours.

Nurses sometimes wonder whether it is good for a child to be visited because he cries when his mother has to go away again. Would it not be better to spare him the tears by not letting her visit at all?

Studies have shown that it is better for the child to be visited, even if he cries after each visit, than that he should be 'good' and alone. The child who cries can be comforted and he soon learns that his mother will come back. The quiet child is keeping all his grief to himself. He thinks his mother has abandoned him, and this is the most dreadful thing that can happen in a child's world. A quiet child is a sick child, either physically or emotionally—or both.

WARD ROUTINE

Because the healthy child is noisy, active and adventurous, a children's ward cannot be run quite like one for adults. Beds will be untidy, toys will be strewn about, children as they get better will be in and out of bed—and under and over them too at times. Although a certain amount of law and order is necessary for everyone's peace of mind, the nurse should let the children have as much freedom as possible. The school teacher and the occupational therapist will keep them interested and occupied for part of the day, while hospitals which allow open visiting find that parents are a great help, not only in playing with the children but at meal times and bed time too. They can help with the routine feeding and washing, leaving the nurse more time for special treatments.

The study of sick children is a very specialized one, and this section touches only the fringe of the subject. Its object is simply to point out some of the ways in which the nursing of children differs from that of adults. Imagination and understanding are part of good nursing in every ward, but especially so in the children's ward, because the sick child is so vulnerable.

20

Special Departments in the Hospital

There are several special departments of the hospital about which the pupil nurse must have some knowledge.

THE X-RAY DEPARTMENT

This is where the photographs are taken which show up the bones and, in many cases, various internal organs and tissues. The taking of X-ray photographs is a very specialized and important job. Patients are many and radiographers are busy people; they have to work to a strict timetable, and yet be ready as well to X-ray casualties who may arrive at any time. So it can be seen that if a patient is being sent from a ward, which is not very far away, it is only fair, as well as courteous, to see that your patient is in the department at the right time. If there is some hold-up which cannot be avoided, such as the patient being sick or a doctor arriving to see him, let the radiographer know at once so that she can get on with something else.

Your patients may need some assurance that nothing dreadful is going to happen. Sometimes the nurse is asked to stay and help if the patient is very heavy or ill. In that case you will be given protective clothing to shield your body from radiation.

For many abdominal X-ray examinations special preparations have to be undertaken for a day or two beforehand in order to

clear the bowel of faeces or gas. Instructions will be sent to the
ward about such things as diet, aperients, enemas, etc., and it is
most important that these orders should be carried out exactly
or the whole thing will have to be done again.

In some hospitals radiation therapy is given as treatment for
cancer and a few other conditions. This may make the patient
feel rather sick and depressed at first, but he can be assured that
this is usual and will soon pass. The skin over these areas must
be treated very gently and have nothing applied to it.

THE OCCUPATIONAL THERAPY DEPARTMENT

This is where a number of patients go for what is called
rehabilitation. If you think about this long word carefully you
can see that it means making people fit for life outside again—to
return to their old habits and place of living once more.

Many of the patients are those who have had some illness or
accident which has deprived them of the use of one or more
limbs, as after a stroke or some other type of paralysis, after a
bad fracture when a limb has not been used for a long time, or
after burns, or neglected arthritis, when the fingers have become
bent and useless.

Here, while their muscles are being re-educated, or new ways
are being found to move helpless fingers or arms, they are also
learning new and pleasant crafts and occupations that may help
them to earn a living outside. They are supplied with all sorts
of gadgets to make life easier, such as long tongs for picking
things up from the floor, cutlery and pencils with handles
fitted with rubber jackets to make them easy to hold, even
devices to enable them to put on their own shoes and stockings,
a feat they may have thought they could never perform again.
Housewives are taught to prepare vegetables and cook in
specially equipped kitchens with utensils that can easily be used
in their own homes. All the time crafts are being taught to
other patients, some still confined to bed, so that basketry,
weaving, rug making and other interesting hobbies help to pass
the otherwise weary hours pleasantly and profitably.

The Patient in Hospital

THE PHYSIOTHERAPY DEPARTMENT

Like the Occupational Therapy department, this one is concerned with getting the patient on his feet again and prepared for an active life. In many ways the two professions work closely together. Here quite strenuous physical exercises may be carried out. Patients are taught to walk again after months in bed. In hospitals dealing with young people who have had polio there is usually a pool where they are first taught to use their limbs by swimming and exercises in water.

All forms of electrical treatment are done here, including infra-red and ultra-violet ray exposure. Massage, which should be attempted only by a qualified physiotherapist, is carried out, and you will often see them in the wards teaching patients to breathe properly or strengthening their muscles before they are to get up for the first time.

THE MEDICAL SOCIAL WORKER'S OFFICE

The medical social worker's office is the centre to which many patients go with problems of all sorts. The medical social workers have been trained in Social Service and it is they who find baby sitters for women who have had to leave their children in a hurry, look for Homes for old people who can leave hospital but have nowhere to go, arrange the transfer of some patients who need different treatment in another hospital, know how to get financial aid for a man who is worried about being out of work, and go out to see the homes and relations of in-patients, to find out for themselves what these people's problems are. These are just a few of the helpful things that are done by medical social workers to make the life of our patients happier by removing personal worries from their minds.

Anatomy and Physiology

21

Anatomy and Physiology: What it Means

Cells and Tissues

The human body is made up of chemicals. Examples of chemicals are oxygen, iron, calcium, iodine, and there are many others. These chemicals are grouped together into millions of tiny units called *cells*.

When the life of a human being begins it starts from a single cell which is formed by the union of a male with a female cell. This fertilized cell divides and multiplies to form the various *tissues* which will have to do different jobs in the body—skin tissues, nerve tissues, muscle tissues and so on.

The tissues group together to form *organs*, for example the stomach, the heart or the brain, each with its own special function to carry out, but all working smoothly together to make the living body.

The cells vary in their shape and general appearance according to the type of tissue they form. A typical cell has a nucleus which is essential to its life and from which it can reproduce other cells, and it will have some or all of the following functions:

1. The power to take up and use nourishment and oxygen
2. The power to get rid of waste matter
3. The power to reproduce itself, by division

4. The power to receive and react to stimuli such as light, heat, etc.
5. The power of movement

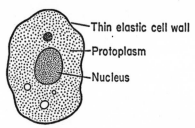

FIG. 13. DIAGRAM OF A TYPICAL CELL

After we are born this process of cell division still goes on until we are fully grown.

In adult life, although we are not growing any bigger, our cells are continually being worn out by the business of living. To keep pace with the wear and tear old cells must be removed and new ones must grow in their place. Our whole body is constantly renewing itself day by day and this ceaseless activity goes on throughout our lives.

As we approach old age the cells begin to lose their power to reproduce themselves and gradually the body falls into disrepair, until finally it can no longer support life, and dies.

Anatomy is the science of the structure of the body and the relationships between its parts.

Physiology deals with the working of the body and the functions of its various organs.

Descriptive Terms

Certain descriptive terms are used in anatomy. These are:

Superior, or upper
Inferior, or lower
Anterior, or front
Posterior, or behind

External, or outside
Internal, or inside
Lateral, or away from the middle line; at the side
Medial, or nearer to the middle line
Median, situated in the middle
Distal, or furthest from the head
Proximal, or nearest to the head

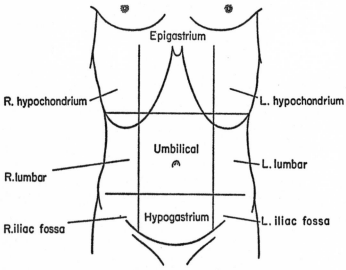

FIG. 14. REGIONS OF THE ABDOMEN

The abdomen is divided into nine regions for describing the exact position of an organ. The nurse may hear these mentioned sometimes, as when a patient suffering from appendicitis is said to have a pain in the right iliac fossa.

SIGNS AND SYMPTOMS

There is quite a difference between the meanings of these two words. _Signs_ are those things you see by looking at a person, the things a doctor is searching for with all his tests. Often the patient does not notice them himself.

Symptoms are the things the patient himself complains of; the ones that sent him to the doctor in the first place, e.g. he has a headache, and says so. Now you cannot see a headache, so that is a symptom. But you may look at a patient and think how red his face is, or how blue his fingers look. But redness or blueness cannot be felt, so they are *signs*.

If a patient is unconscious, there can only be signs because he will not be able to say what he is feeling.

22

The Framework of the Body: The Skeletal System

Bone when fully developed consists of one-third animal matter—cells, blood vessels and a gelatinous substance called *collagen*—and two-thirds mineral matter, *calcium* and *phosphorus*. In young children the animal matter is greater, so the bones are softer. The minerals are deposited over the years, until in old people the bones are much harder and more fragile, thus breaking more easily.

If you cut across a bone you will see that the outer part is very dense, like ivory. This is called *compact* tissue. Nearer the middle it looks much looser, rather like a honeycomb. This is called *cancellous* tissue (think of lots of little cells).

Right in the centre is a space filled with marrow. This hollow makes the bones much lighter than if they were solid, and Nature has used this space as a factory to make both red and white blood cells. In growing children all the bones have these factories, but by adult life when less new blood is required, most of the 'red' marrow turns to fat or 'yellow' marrow, and only the upper ends of the femur and humerus, and the flat bones, go on turning out blood cells.

Except at the ends, each bone is covered with a membrane known as *periosteum*. Tiny blood vessels pierce the bone beneath this covering and communicate with a system of

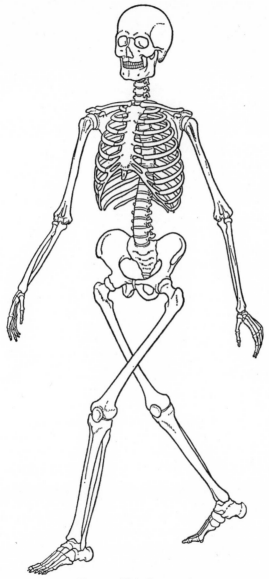

FIG. 15. THE SKELETON

195

minute canals which permit the circulation of blood through the bone. The ends of long bones are covered with *hyaline cartilage,* a specially tough tissue which protects the parts which receive most pressure.

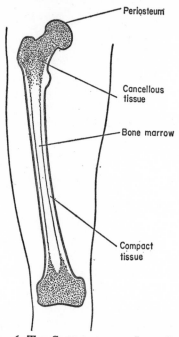

FIG. 16. THE STRUCTURE OF A LONG BONE

After a bone has been broken, if the parts are brought together properly and kept in a good position, blood and lymph bring salts and other things needed for repair. Each edge then begins to throw out new cells which grow out to meet those coming from the other broken parts. In the end they all meet and join up, and the break is healed. This lump of new bone is called *callus,* and the bone may even be stronger than it was before the accident.

Bones are classified as:

Long, e.g. the bones of the arm and leg
Short, e.g. those of the wrist and foot
Flat, e.g. skull, sternum, shoulder blades
Irregular, e.g. the bones of the spine (vertebrae)

The skeleton is made up of the *skull,* the *bones* of the *thorax* or *chest,* the *backbone* or *vertebral column,* the *pelvis,* and the *bones* of the *limbs* and *hands* and *feet.*

There is a special way to describe bones. The long part is called the *shaft,* and the various knobs and points are called *processes, condyles, trochanters* and so on.

The Skull

The skull consists of the *cranium* which protects the brain, and the bones of the face. The roof and sides of the cranial cavity

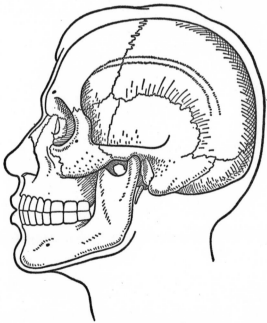

FIG. 17. SIDE VIEW OF THE SKULL

197

form the *vault* of the skull; the floor of the cavity is referred to as the *base* of the skull.

The skull is made up of many bones which are joined together to form immovable joints. In an infant, however, the bones at the top of the head are not completely joined. The spaces between them are called *fontanelles* and can be felt through the scalp. They gradually close up as the bones grow.

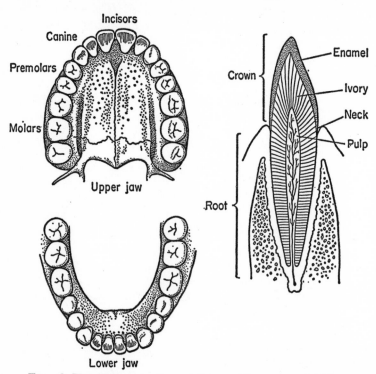

FIG. 18. THE UPPER AND LOWER SETS OF TEETH, AND (*right*) A
SECTION THROUGH A TYPICAL TOOTH

The teeth are contained in sockets in the spongy parts of the upper and lower jaws.

Each tooth consists of a *root*, a *crown* and a *neck*, and is made up of *ivory* or *dentine* which gives shape to the tooth, and encloses a pulp cavity containing nerves and blood vessels. *Enamel*, the hardest substance in the body, caps the crown.

The teeth begin to form before birth and the temporary or milk teeth come through from about six months onwards.

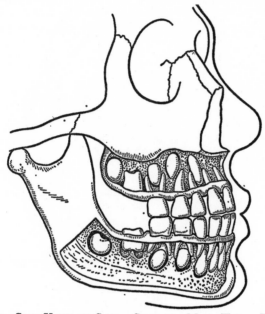

FIG. 19. SIDE VIEW OF SKULL SHOWING MILK TEETH ERUPTED AND PERMANENT TEETH IN JAW ABOVE AND BELOW

The *temporary* teeth are replaced by the *permanent* teeth between the sixth and twelfth year, with the exception of the last molars or wisdom teeth, which do not appear until between the seventeenth and twenty-fifth year and often much later.

Sinuses are hollow spaces. There are several such spaces in the head, which are filled with air and lined with a mucous membrane which is continuous with that lining the nose. They make the bones lighter and give tone and volume to the voice. We appreciate their value when they become blocked, as when we have a cold. These sinuses open into the nose and the nasopharynx and are liable to cause great discomfort if they become inflamed. This condition is called *sinusitis*.

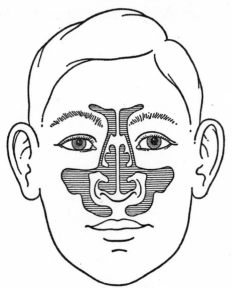

FIG. 20. THE PARANASAL SINUSES, FRONT VIEW

The Thorax

The bones of the thorax are:

The Sternum. A flat, dagger-shaped bone in front of the chest.

The Ribs. Twelve flat, curved bones. They are attached to the vertebrae behind and to the sternum in front, with the exception of the last two which are only attached to the vertebrae and so are called 'floating' ribs.

The Spinal Column

The spinal column is a flexible structure supporting the head and protecting the spinal cord. It consists of vertebrae and intervertebral discs.

THE VERTEBRAE

There are thirty-three vertebrae. These are divided into:

7 cervical (or neck) vertebrae
12 thoracic vertebrae
5 lumbar vertebrae
5 sacral vertebrae (fused into the sacrum in an adult)
4 coccygeal vertebrae (fused into the coccyx in an adult)

A vertebra consists of a body, an arch and seven processes.

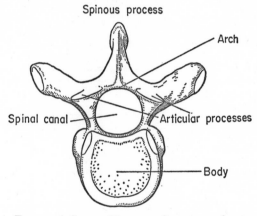

Spinous process

Arch

Spinal canal

Articular processes

Body

FIG. 21. A SIMPLE VERTEBRA SEEN FROM ABOVE

The arch is formed by two processes which project backwards on either side of the body, and then continue backwards as the spinous process.

The articular processes form joints with the vertebrae above and below.

When the vertebrae are joined together their arches form the spinal canal, through which the spinal cord passes.

INTERVERTEBRAL DISCS

Between the bodies of the vertebrae are discs of cartilage which act as buffers in counteracting shock and give freedom of movement. If one of these discs is damaged it can press on surrounding nerves and cause pain and backache according to the region affected, a condition commonly known today as a 'slipped disc'. These discs separate the vertebrae and allow a

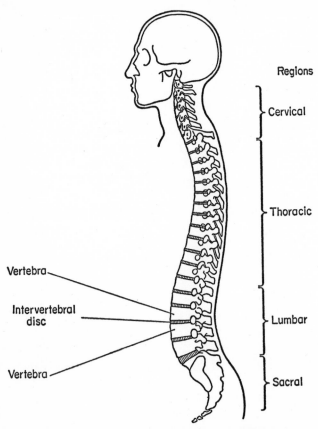

Regions

Cervical

Thoracic

Vertebra

Intervertebral
disc

Lumbar

Vertebra

Sacral

FIG. 22. THE SPINAL COLUMN SHOWING INTERVERTEBRAL DISCS
AND LUMBAR CURVE

limited power of rotation and slight movement backwards, forwards and from side to side.

The column bends forward in the cervical and lumbar regions and backward in the thoracic and sacral.

The Shoulder Girdle

The shoulder girdle supports the upper limbs and consists of the *clavicle* (collar bone) and *scapula* (shoulder blade) on each side. The *clavicle* is a long bone with a double curve, lying above the first rib. It articulates with the sternum and with the scapula. The *scapula* is a large, flat, triangular bone placed on the back of the thorax.

The Bones of the Upper Limb

The *humerus* is a long bone, with a head which fits into a shallow cup on the scapula and a shaft which ends in two condyles for articulation with the bones of the forearm. The upper part of the shaft of the humerus is sometimes called the *surgical neck* because it is the part which is most easily broken.

The *forearm* consists of two bones, the radius and the ulna. The *radius* is on the thumb side of the arm. Here we can take the pulse most easily, as the radial artery passes over it quite near the skin. The *ulna*, the upper end of which forms the prominence of the elbow, is on the little finger side.

The wrists or *carpal bones* consist of eight small irregular bones arranged in two rows.

The *palm* of the hand is made up of five *metacarpal* bones, and the *fingers* of fourteen *phalanges,* three in each finger and two in the thumb.

The Pelvis

The pelvis is made up of the two hip bones, or *innominate* bones, the *sacrum* and the *coccyx*.

The two *innominate* bones are composed of the *ilium,* the

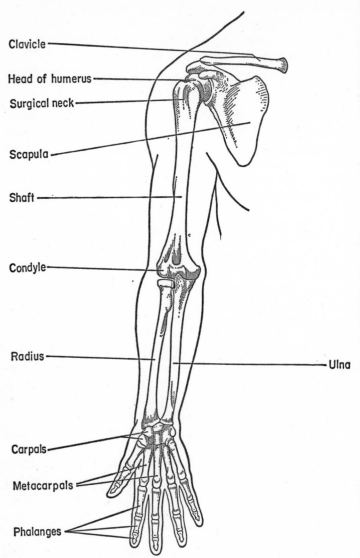

Clavicle

Head of humerus

Surgical neck

Scapula

Shaft

Condyle

Radius

Ulna

Carpals

Metacarpals

Phalanges

FIG. 23. THE BONES OF THE UPPER LIMB

broad expanded part of the hip; the *ischium,* the lower and stronger portion which supports the body when seated, and the *pubis,* the front and most slender part. These bones fuse together at the side to form a cup-like depression known as the *acetabulum* which holds the head of the femur.

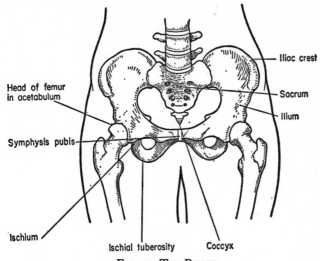

FIG. 24. THE PELVIS

The female pelvis is wider, and its inside cavity is larger than that of the male, because of its importance in pregnancy.

The Bones of the Lower Limb

The *femur* or *thigh bone* is the longest, strongest and heaviest bone in the body. Its head fits into the acetabulum and forms the hip joint. The shaft ends in two large bony condyles.

The condyles of the femur articulate with the *tibia* or inner bone of the leg to form the knee joint, and the *patella,* or knee cap lies over the joint in the tendon of the thigh muscle. The tibia has a sharp ridge, the shin, which, since it is unprotected by muscles, can be felt under the skin.

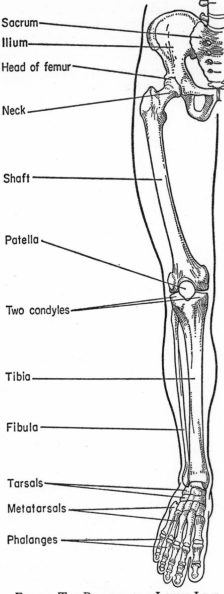

Sacrum

Ilium

Head of femur

Neck

Shaft

Patella

Two condyles

Tibia

Fibula

Tarsals

Metatarsals

Phalanges

FIG. 25. THE BONES OF THE LOWER LIMB

The *fibula* or outer bone articulates with the tibia at its upper end and with the foot at the lower end.

These two bones, the tibia and the fibula, are arranged rather like a brooch with its pin.

The bones of the foot consist of seven *tarsal* bones.

Five *metatarsal* bones correspond with the five metacarpal bones in the hand, and the fourteen *phalanges* in the *toes* are similar to those in the *fingers*.

THE ARCHES OF THE FOOT

The arches of the foot support the weight of the body and are formed as a result of:

1. The shape and arrangement of the bones
2. The tension or pull of the ligaments
3. The muscles and faciae in the sole of the foot

There are two *longitudinal* arches and one *transverse* arch.

Sometimes these arches drop, causing the feet to ache badly. This is the condition known as *flat foot*. It is produced by certain weakening illnesses, by jobs involving a great deal of walking or standing, especially if the subject walks badly, or by wearing the wrong kind of shoes. The foot should always be placed straight, and not allowed to turn outwards, so that the body weight is evenly distributed along its length.

The Joints

A *joint* is an *articulation*, that is a meeting point of two or more bones.

THE CHIEF KINDS OF JOINT

Fibrous or immovable. Found in the skull as the sutures
Cartilaginous or slightly movable. Found between the bones of
the spinal column and pelvis

Synovial or freely movable. Found in the limbs

In slightly movable joints the bones are separated by a pad of cartilage. In freely movable joints the ends of the bones are also separated by cartilage and the whole joint is surrounded by a

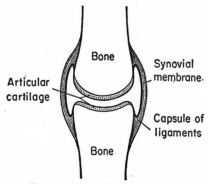

FIG. 26. DIAGRAM OF A FREELY MOVABLE JOINT

capsule or covering of ligaments and lined by a special membrane which secretes synovial fluid. This fluid 'oils' the joint so that it moves easily. The ligaments are like ropes lashing the bones together in such a way that they can move only in the proper direction.

A sprain is due to a ligament getting torn while trying to keep the bones in their right position when we twist or wrench a joint. If they fail to hold, the joint may be torn right out of its proper position; this is called a dislocation.

There are several varieties of freely movable joints, for example:

1. *Ball and socket,* where a head fits into a cup-shaped socket, e.g. the shoulder and hip.

2. *Pivot,* where one bone turns on another, e.g. the radius on the ulna when the wrist is turned.

3. *Hinge,* where a limb is able to bend and straighten itself, e.g. the elbow and the knee.

4. *Gliding,* where the surface of one bone moves over the surface of another, e.g. the bones of the hand and foot.

Bursae are closed sacs containing fluid, which protect a joint from pressure. e.g. the bursae over the knee joint.

Certain definite movements take place at joints. These are:

1. *Flexion,* or bending.
2. *Extension,* or straightening.
3. *Adduction,* or movement towards the middle line.
4. *Abduction,* or movement away from the middle line.
5. *Circumduction,* or movement of the limb in a circle.
6. *External rotation,* or turning outwards from the middle line.
7. *Internal rotation,* or turning inwards towards the middle line.
8. *Supination,* or turning the palm of the hand to face upwards.
9. *Pronation,* or turning the palm downwards.

The best way to learn these movements is to practise them with your own arm or leg and watch what is happening.

THE BONES IN THE PRINCIPAL JOINTS OF THE BODY

The shoulder. Scapula and humerus
The elbow. Humerus, radius and ulna
The wrist. Radius and three carpal bones
The hip. Innominate bone and femur
The knee. Femur, tibia and patella
The ankle. Tibia, fibula and talus

Some Disorders of the Bones and Joints

Acute rheumatism (Rheumatic fever)

This is a disease of young people. It usually follows a sore throat, and can lead to heart disease in later life. There is a high temperature, and the joints become tender, red and swollen, one after another. The child feels very ill. He needs very good and gentle nursing to prevent the heart becoming affected.

Arthritis

This is inflammation of the joints.

Rheumatoid arthritis affects quite young people and is a very crippling and painful condition with general illness as well. The drug cortisone helps to control it, though it does not cure. Radiation therapy (treatment with special rays) helps some patients.

Osteo-arthritis usually occurs later in life. It affects only the joints. The ends of the bones in the joint become rough and jagged so that any movement hurts. The patient is not ill in himself. Sometimes the surgeon will operate on the joints to stop the surfaces rubbing together, and so relieve the pain.

Bursitis

Inflammation of a bursa, i.e. one of the sacs filled with synovial fluid situated between the movable parts of a joint. Pre-patellar bursitis is 'housemaid's knee'.

Osteomyelitis

This is an infection of bone and marrow caused by germs which produce pus (usually staphylococci). It is not so common as it used to be, but can follow illnesses such as measles, if the child injures himself while he is still very run down. It can also follow any accident in which a bone has been injured and germs have got in through the damaged periosteum. It is a very painful disease, and may destroy parts of the bone, but treatment with modern drugs, such as penicillin, and good nursing cure most cases.

Paget's disease

This occurs in elderly people, and may be seen in geriatric wards. No one knows the cause, but the bones become thin and brittle, with various deformities, and break easily. Great care must be taken when bathing such patients or helping them to get up so that they do not fall.

23

Movement: The Muscular System

The muscular system is responsible for the movements of the body.

The *voluntary muscles* which are attached to the limbs are so called because they are under the control of the will.

Muscles end in tendons, cords of varying length and thickness, by means of which they are attached to the end of bones in a broad sheath of fibrous tissue which helps to protect the organs underneath.

As a result of nerve stimulation, muscles have the power of contracting and then relaxing again. The energy which enables them to work, comes from the burning up in the body of foodstuffs, mainly carbohydrates, from which glucose, the main fuel of the body, is produced.

Muscular activity is the result of a complicated series of chemical reactions for which glucose and oxygen brought to the muscles in the blood stream are essential. Therefore, muscular effort is dependent upon an adequate food supply and a good circulation.

Many muscles are arranged in pairs and oppose each other in action; this occurs where the arm is bent at the elbow by means of the biceps muscle, which is inserted just below the head of the radius, and straightened by means of the triceps, which lies on the back of the upper arm and is inserted into the point of the elbow.

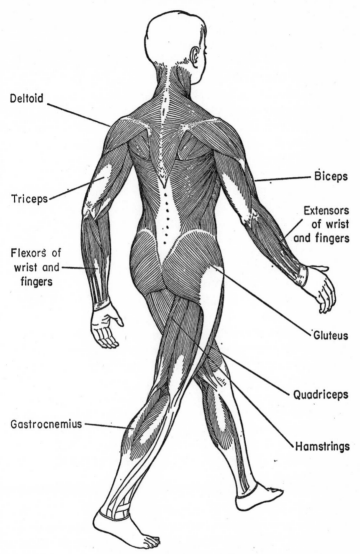

FIG. 27. THE MUSCULAR SYSTEM

The deltoid lies over the shoulder and lifts the arm away from the body (abducts). It can be used as a site for giving intramuscular injections.

The body is raised on the toes through the action of the muscles of the gastrocnemius which is inserted behind the ankle joint into the point of the heel.

The buttocks are formed by a pair of very strong muscles called the gluteus maximus muscles, which enable us to stand up, and to run and walk. These muscles are sometimes used as the site for injections (p. 101); in giving these, however, great care must be used because a great nerve, the sciatic nerve, runs just underneath gluteus maximus.

In front of the thigh is a big four-part muscle called the quadriceps, which straightens the knee. The quadriceps is a safe site for injections. Down the back of the thigh run the hamstrings, which bend the knee.

The skull is covered with a sheet of muscle which is attached to the occipital bone and inserted into the tissues above the eyebrows, lifting the forehead and drawing the scalp backwards. The tongue too is a muscle, probably the hardest worked of all except the heart.

The muscles of the face are responsible for the movements of the eyes, the eyelids, for mastication and for speech.

The wonderful movements of the hand are performed by no fewer than twenty-seven bones and twenty-eight muscles. Fortunately the nurse does not need to know all their names. The muscles that bend the fingers are called *flexors* and those that straighten them are called *extensors*.

The diaphragm is the dome-shaped muscle which divides the chest from the abdomen. It forms the floor of the former and the roof of the latter.

In breathing, it contracts and flattens, so enlarging the chest cavity so that the lungs can expand and take in more air (inspiration). When it relaxes, it rises up again and pushes the air out (expiration). This movement is repeated about 20 times a minute all through life.

The diaphragm is one of the most important muscles in the

body. When it is paralysed, as sometimes happens, for example, in poliomyelitis, the patient has to be nursed with the help of a respirator to enable him to breathe.

It also helps in actions requiring downward pressure, such as opening the bowels and passing urine, and in childbirth.

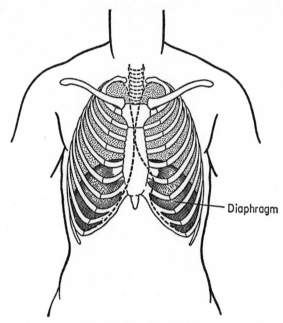

FIG. 28. THE DIAPHRAGM

Involuntary muscles are found in organs such as the intestines, stomach, bladder and uterus, and are not under the control of the will. These muscles produce different movements from those of the external ones. These include:

(a) Peristalsis which passes food on its way (p. 241).
(b) The special rhythmic contractions which we call the beating of the heart.

The involuntary muscles go on working even while we are asleep or unconscious.

Disorders of the Muscular System

Fibrositis. This is what we often think of as 'rheumatism'. It is inflammation of connective tissues round muscles and joints. Heat and massage help to relieve the pain and stiffness.

Muscular dystrophy and *myasthenia gravis* are diseases in which the muscles gradually lose their power until the patient is quite helpless.

24

The Body's Transport System: The Circulatory and Lymphatic Systems

The circulatory system consists of the heart, the blood vessels and the blood.

The Heart

The heart is a hollow, muscular organ about the size of its owner's clenched fist. It lies in the chest, between the lungs, pointing downwards towards the left. The base or wider end lies behind the centre of the sternum, and the apex or pointed end rests on the diaphragm, in the space between the fifth and sixth ribs.

The heart, which weighs about 10 ounces, is divided into two distinct halves by a wall called the *septum*. These halves have no communication with each other after birth. In the rare cases where the prenatal (before birth) communication continues into childhood, circulation of oxygen-bearing blood is hampered and in some forms of this congenital type of heart disease the infant is cyanosed from birth and therefore often referred to as a 'blue baby'. Each side of the heart is divided again into two chambers, an upper one, the *atrium*, which receives the blood and a lower one, the *ventricle,* which discharges the blood. Each

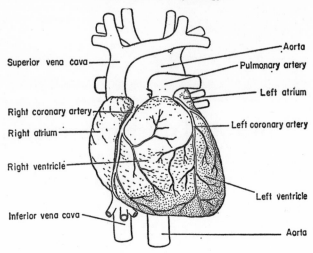

Aorta

Pulmonary artery

Left atrium

Superior vena cava

Right coronary artery

Right atrium

Left coronary artery

Right ventricle

Left ventricle

Inferior vena cava

Aorta

FIG. 29. THE HEART

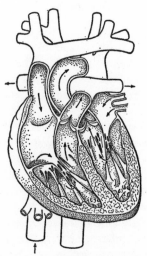

FIG. 30. INTERIOR OF THE HEART SHOWING DIRECTION
OF BLOOD FLOW

atrium opens into the corresponding ventricle by an opening which is guarded by a valve.

The valve on the right side is called the *tricuspid valve,* because it has three cusps or flaps, and that on the left is called the *mitral valve,* because, having two cusps, it is thought to look like a bishop's mitre.

The heart is like two pumps placed side by side. The one on the left has much stronger, thicker walls, because it has to pump the blood much further than the one on the right. The pump on the right only sends the returned (de-oxygenated) blood into the lungs to get some more oxygen. The pump on the left sends the blood all round the body.

CIRCULATION THROUGH THE HEART

Blood from which oxygen has been used up, coming from all parts of the body, is collected into two big veins, the *superior* and *inferior venae cavae,* which empty into the right atrium. From here it is pumped into the right ventricle, which contracts and drives it into the lungs to pick up more oxygen.

Oxygenated blood is then brought back to the left atrium. From here it passes into the left ventricle, which contracts and drives it into the biggest artery in the body, the *aorta.* This great vessel gives off many branches which eventually take the blood to all parts of the body.

The heart muscle itself must be supplied with blood. This comes from the important coronary arteries, which encircle the heart like a crown.

DISORDERS OF THE HEART

Angina

This is a condition caused by the gradual narrowing of the coronary arteries, the arteries supplying the heart muscle itself. The sufferer has attacks of cramp-like pain up the left side of his chest, neck, and left arm. Drugs such as amyl nitrite and glyceryl trinitrate control these attacks, as long as the patient lives a very quiet life.

Congestive heart failure

In this condition the blood does not flow properly. It stays too long in the lungs, so fluid seeps through the capillaries and blocks up some of the air sacs, and breathing becomes difficult *(dyspnoea)*. It stays too long in the tissues, and the body gets swollen with fluid *(oedema)*. Fluid fills up spaces in the abdomen *(ascites)*, and pressure on the stomach may cause bleeding *(haematemesis)*.

All this sounds very alarming, and the patient is, indeed, very ill, but with the treatments given today a great improvement can take place. The fluid can be removed by drainage. The heart can be made to beat more strongly by the drug *digitalis*. The kidneys can move extra fluid with the help of other drugs. A special diet without salt is given, because salt tends to hold the fluid back. Oxygen will help breathing, and with complete rest the patient gradually improves. He can often go home and live a normal life if he is very careful.

Coronary thrombosis

This condition may occur if a clot of blood is formed in these diseased arteries and gets stuck, cutting off the life-giving oxygen to the heart. If the clot, known as a thrombus, is a big one, the patient dies at once. If some blood can get through he may recover after a long period of rest; drugs, such as heparin, are given in order to stop any more clotting.

Embolism

An embolism is a clot that has formed and is moving round the blood vessels. It can get stuck in the lungs *(pulmonary embolism)*, and may cause sudden death or destruction of some of the lung tissue. It may lodge in the brain *(cerebral embolism)* and cause a stroke or apoplexy.

An embolus is a moving clot. A thrombus is one that has got

held up in a vessel. The amount of damage it does depends on where it is.

Endocarditis and Pericarditis

These conditions are inflammation of either the lining or the covering of the heart. They are both complications of some earlier infection. The commonest cause is rheumatic fever, or an infection by some variety of the germ called streptococcus. Endocarditis is the more serious since the valves are involved and, because these control the flow of blood through the heart, the whole circulation is affected, so every part of the body must suffer in time. With good nursing, and the use of antibiotics, the patient usually gets well enough to lead a fairly normal life. Many years later, however, he may get the condition known as congestive heart failure.

The Blood Vessels

Arteries are vessels carrying blood away from the heart, and, with the exception of the pulmonary artery, carry oxygenated

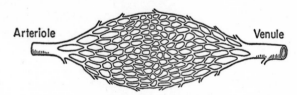

Fig. 31. A Capillary Network, where Artery and Vein meet

blood. Since they have to stretch with each beat of the heart the walls of the arteries have a good deal of elastic tissue in them. As they reach the tissues the arteries divide into smaller vessels called arterioles.

Veins are vessels carrying blood back to the heart. They are thinner and less elastic than arteries, and those of the limbs have valves all the way up because the blood has to pass in an upward direction. The smallest veins are called venules.

Capillaries are the smallest vessels of all, and connect the arteries with the veins. They are found all over the body.

The *pulse* is the wave of movement which passes along the wall of an artery each time the heart beats. It is best felt where an artery passes over a bone, e.g. the radial artery at the wrist.

Blood pressure means the amount of pressure of the blood against the wall of an artery. It varies with the condition of the heart, the amount of blood in the body, the state of the artery walls, and the size of the capillaries.

It is an important guide in certain diseases, and is measured with an instrument called a *sphygmomanometer.*

The Blood

The blood is a sticky fluid with a salty taste. It is composed of red blood cells, white blood cells, platelets and a fluid, plasma. There are about 6 litres or 10 pints of it in the body.

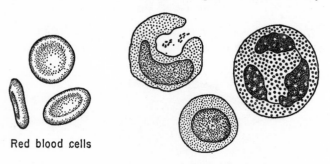

Red blood cells

White blood cells

Fig. 32

Red blood cells are little discs with depressions on each side. There are about five million in every cubic millimetre of blood. They are so small that seventy-five thousand million of them could fit into a 1-inch cube! They contain an iron-rich substance called *haemoglobin,* which combines with oxygen in the lungs. It is this function of being able to carry oxygen which makes the red blood cells of such supreme importance to life.

Lack of iron to make haemoglobin is one of the commonest causes of anaemia.

The red blood cells are made in the bone-marrow. They live for about 7 to 12 weeks, and are then destroyed by special cells in the spleen. The iron left over is used again for new red blood cells.

White blood cells are irregular in shape and much larger than the red. Their main function is to fight infection by devouring germs which may enter the body. At such times they multiply very rapidly, doubling or trebling their average number of 7,000 per cubic millimetre. Some are made in the spleen and some in the bone-marrow.

There are several types with long names that you may see in a 'differential blood count'. This is important to the doctor because the presence of abnormal numbers of some of these cells may help him with a diagnosis.

Platelets are the smallest cells of all, and number 300,000 per cubic millimetre. Their function is to aid the clotting of blood when injury occurs, because they contain a special substance that is only released when it is needed. A clot 'stops up' an injured blood vessel like a cork, and so prevents more blood escaping.

Plasma is the liquid part of the blood in which float the blood cells. It is made up of water, all the food substances after digestion, waste matter being taken to the kidneys or skin, secretions from the glands, gases like oxygen and carbon dioxide, and protective substances which help the body to overcome infection or prevent haemorrhage. Plasma also contains proteins, which are responsible for the stickiness of the blood and play an important part in regulating the amount of water that leaves the blood through the capillary walls.

(Serum, a term you will often hear used, is plasma with the proteins removed so that it cannot clot.)

THE CLOTTING OF BLOOD

Clotting occurs normally only in injury, in order to prevent or stop bleeding. It is brought about by several substances found in the plasma reacting with another substance found in the platelets, and a clot is formed at the mouth of the bleeding vessel, acting like a plug.

THE FUNCTIONS OF THE BLOOD

1. To carry oxygen and food to the tissues.
2. To carry waste products to the organs which excrete them.
3. To carry secretions from the glands to where they are wanted.
4. To seal wounds by its power of clotting.
5. To protect from infection.
6. To maintain the normal temperature of the body.
7. To carry water to the tissues.

DISORDERS OF THE BLOOD AND VESSELS

Anaemia

This is an impoverished state of the blood. There are several causes. The red blood cells may be too few or undeveloped. They may not be able to carry enough haemoglobin. Blood may have been lost by bleeding, as in childbirth or accident, or from piles or heavy periods; or the substances necessary for making blood may be missing from the diet.

Such patients look pale, get very tired and breathless if they make any effort. Their ankles may swell. They will get indigestion and headaches and be very irritable. The cause has to be found and then treated with extra vitamins, perhaps B_{12}, and drugs such as iron are given, together with good diet, rest, and sometimes blood transfusions.

Leukaemia

This is a form of cancer of the tissues that make some of the white cells (leucocytes). They increase so much that the red ones are crowded out so that there are not enough to carry

oxygen. It is, unhappily, a disease which can occur in children
and young adults. Treatment, particularly blood transfusions,
can make the patient feel more comfortable, but there is as yet
no cure.

Arteriosclerosis

This means hardening of the arteries (*sclera* means hard,
dense). A change in the artery walls takes place, making them
less elastic and even chalky. The blood cannot flow so evenly,
and the blood pressure goes up, sometimes to dangerous levels.
The patient has severe headaches, cramps, changes in vision
and many other symptoms.

Varicose veins are ones which have become weak and flabby.
They swell with the blood which they are not capable of sending
back to the heart. They occur in the legs, and as piles (haemorrhoids) in the rectum. They occur in people who have to stand
for long periods, or where there is much pressure from above, as
in pregnancy or chronic constipation.

The Lymphatic System

Lymph is a colourless fluid derived from the blood, which
passes from the capillaries into the cells of the body. From the
tissues it is collected into small vessels called *lymph vessels* or
lymphatics, which begin in spaces between the cells and unite
to form larger vessels which run side by side with the blood
vessels, both near the surface and deep down. Eventually they
all drain into two large ducts which pour the lymph into the
blood stream at the root of the neck.

Lymph glands are found along the course of the lymphatics,
some in the groin, under the arm, in the neck, and in the pelvic
and abdominal cavities. They help to keep back germs which
might otherwise enter the blood stream. Sometimes they
become swollen, showing that they have done this successfully.
The tonsils are extra large lymphatic glands.

The *spleen* is the largest lymphatic gland of all. It lies to the left of the stomach and is about 5 inches long. It is soft and purple, and holds a lot of blood. (Damage to it is a frequent cause of internal haemorrhage in road accidents.)

Its functions are:

1. To destroy old red blood cells and send the useful bits back to the liver to be used again.
2. To make some of the white cells.
3. To make some of the substances called antibodies that protect us against diseases.

DISORDERS OF LYMPH GLANDS

Tonsillitis

This is the commonest disorder of a lymphatic gland. Having done their work of filtering the lymph and stopping unwelcome visitors like streptococci from entering the blood stream, the tonsils themselves become so full of them that they become very inflamed and painful. If pus forms we call the condition a quinsy and the abscess may have to be opened.

Hot gargles, plenty of fluids, soothing lozenges, kaolin poultices to the neck (heat is always comforting), injections of penicillin and rest in bed while the temperature is high are the usual lines of treatment.

If, after several such attacks, it is decided that the tonsils are no longer able to do their work properly, the doctor may advise their removal (tonsillectomy).

Hodgkin's Disease

Like leukaemia, this disease is a kind of cancer, but affecting the lymph glands all over the body. This condition, too, affects young people and is at present incurable. A great deal of research is being done by scientists on these two diseases, and there is always hope that one day the cause and cure will be found.

25

How We Breathe:
The Respiratory System

The respiratory system consists of the *nose*, the *larynx*, the *trachea*, the *bronchi* and the *lungs*.

The *nose*, the organ of smell, is a triangular framework of bone and cartilage covered by skin and lined with mucous membrane. The nostrils are provided with short hairs which filter dust from the air. Blood capillaries in the mucous membrane warm the air as it enters, and the mucus helps to moisten it and to trap dust.

The *larynx*, a triangular box-shaped organ which contains the *vocal cords*, lies high up in the front of the neck. The vocal cords produce the sound of the voice.

The larynx is protected above by a leaf-shaped piece of cartilage called the *epiglottis* which prevents food or drink from entering the wind pipe via the larynx and so causing choking.

The *trachea or windpipe* is a tube about $4\frac{1}{2}$ inches long. At the back it rests on the *oesophagus* or food pipe. Just behind the upper end of the sternum it divides into two branches, one for each lung. These are the *bronchi*, which again divide into branches for each lobe of either lung. It is these bronchial tubes which are inflamed in bronchitis. Like the blood vessels they gradually become smaller and smaller until they can be seen only by means of a microscope. Eventually they end as delicate *air sacs* or *alveoli*.

The *lungs* are two cone-shaped spongy organs situated in the chest. They are covered with a double layer of membrane, the *pleura*. Inflammation of this covering is called *pleurisy*.

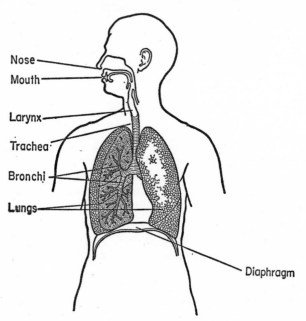

FIG. 33. THE RESPIRATORY SYSTEM

The tiny air sacs are closely surrounded by capillaries, and it is here that fresh oxygen from the air breathed in passes across the cell wall into the blood and the carbon dioxide from the blood passes into the air to be breathed out.

These little air sacs are something like minute bubbles or balloons. They are so tiny that they cannot be seen by the naked eye. Yet there are so many of them that if they were flattened out and joined together they would cover an area thirty times larger than all the skin of the body.

RESPIRATION

Respiration is the act of breathing; it consists of:

Inspiration or the taking in of air. This is the result of the chest enlarging and the lungs expanding. It occurs when the muscles between the ribs lift them, and the diaphragm contracts and flattens. Every time this happens air rushes into the lungs and fills them.

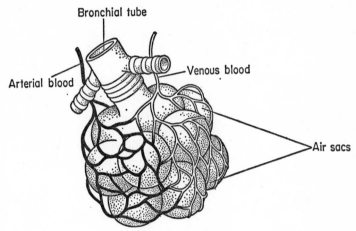

Bronchial tube

Venous blood

Arterial blood

Air sacs

FIG. 34. AIR SACS

Expiration or expelling air from the lungs occurs when all the above muscles relax and the chest returns to its normal size, forcing the air out of the lungs.

All the time the interchange of gases continues in the lungs, oxygen being taken into the red blood cells while carbon dioxide is being given off.

The act of breathing occurs about 18 times per minute in a normal adult, though it is much quicker in a baby.

Air consists mainly of three gases, nitrogen, oxygen and carbon dioxide, and some water vapour. The nitrogen is of no importance here; it is oxygen on which all living things depend. With each breath the blood receives oxygen and gives off carbon dioxide. The latter, however, is not solely a waste material because, while it is in the blood stream, it stimulates the nerve centre in the brain which controls breathing. For this reason the nurse will sometimes see in the ward a carbon dioxide cylinder side by side with an oxygen one, and may see it given to a patient whose breathing is very slow and shallow. The giving of this gas makes the patient breathe more deeply and quickly, thus enabling him to take in more of the life-giving oxygen.

DISORDERS OF THE RESPIRATORY SYSTEM

Asthma

This is a condition in which the bronchial tubes go into a state of spasm, and for a time get so narrow that the sufferer feels as if he was choking. He can breathe in, but cannot get the air out again without a violent struggle which exhausts and frightens him. He is relieved by an injection of adrenaline, but since the cause varies in every case this must be looked into before any satisfactory solution can be found.

Bronchitis

This is inflammation of the bronchial tubes. It occurs during cold, foggy weather, often after a cold. It is not a serious disease at first, but if it comes on too often it becomes chronic, until the patient is never without a cough. In time it can cause damage to the lung tissue.

Bronchiectasis

This is a condition where some of the weak patches in the bronchial tree dilate into sacs or little bags that collect pus which the patient cannot cough up, it is one of the possible results of chronic bronchitis. The patient becomes ill and cannot breathe properly. It is for this condition that you will see postural drainage used.

For *postural drainage* a special bed is used. By turning a
handle the centre is raised so that the patient's head and chest
are lowered so that the foul matter from the base of the lungs
which accumulates in such diseases as bronchiectasis can drain
out into a receiver, so saving the patient the effort of continuous
coughing.

Pleurisy

This means inflammation of the pleura, the covering of the
lungs. It is usually a complication of other diseases such as
tuberculosis or pneumonia. It causes much pain, because the
pleura has to go on moving all the time as the patient breathes,
so it can never rest. Sometimes fluid seeps in between the two
layers of which the pleura is composed. This is 'wet' pleurisy.
It may turn to pus which the doctor will draw off (aspirate)
with a long needle.

The general treatment will be for the underlying cause.

Pneumonia

This is inflammation of another part of the lungs, this time of
the air sacs. It is always caused by bacteria, the most acute type
by the pneumococcus, but several other germs can cause it as
well.

Lobar pneumonia affects one lung at a time, and is commoner
in young adults. *Bronchopneumonia* is scattered about the lungs
in patches, and affects very young children (especially after
measles), and old people.

Treatment includes the use of the most suitable antibiotic
drug, good nursing and oxygen, often concentrated as in an
oxygen tent. This is to load up the blood with extra supplies to
make up for the number of alveoli which are out of action.

26

Food and Nutrition

Food is anything which will provide material for growth and repair of the tissues, and give heat and energy. Most food substances are very complicated and so have to be changed by the digestive processes before they can be absorbed and used by the tissues.

Food is divided into six essential parts with which the body must be supplied every day:

1. PROTEINS

The best of these are found in meat, eggs, milk, fish and cheese, and second class types in peas, beans, lentils and nuts.

Proteins are necessary for growth, especially in the earliest years, and for the repair of tissues after work.

2. CARBOHYDRATES

These are starches and sugars. They are found in bread, potatoes, cereals, flour, honey, fruit, especially grapes, and sugar.

They give the heat and energy to the body.

The simplest form of carbohydrate is called *glucose*, and it is into this that the body changes this type of food before it can be used in the cells.

3. FATS

These are found in animal foods, meat, fish such as herrings and salmon, milk and cream, butter, margarine and oils.

They are chemically very like the carbohydrates, but produce much more heat and energy, so we do not require so much of them.

4. WATER

This is required by the body in large quantities to produce the blood and other body fluids, and for the removal of waste products and to replace all that is lost by the sweat and other excretions. A man can live for two months without food, but only a few days without water.

5. MINERALS

There are many minerals and they are required by the body for a number of purposes. The following are a few examples:

Calcium, found in dairy produce, fish, meat and vegetables, is used by the body to make bones and teeth, and it helps with the clotting of the blood and in ensuring the proper action of the heart and smooth working of the muscles.

Phosphorus is required by the bones, nerves and glands. It is found in dairy produce, oatmeal and meat and fish.

Iron is necessary for the red blood cells. It is found in green vegetables, liver, meat, eggs, dried fruit and cocoa.

Iodine, found in fish, and in vegetables grown near the sea, is necessary for the hormone of the thyroid gland.

6. VITAMINS

These are chemical substances essential for growth and the proper functioning of every part of the body. Much research is continually being done on them and many new ones are being discovered and tested, but basically the following classification may be used:

Vitamin A strengthens resistance to infection. It is essential for healthy membranes, especially of the respiratory tract and eyes. It is found in all dairy produce, fats, cod-liver oil, liver and green vegetables.

Vitamin B has many parts and is referred to as the 'Vitamin B Complex'. One part is essential for the proper formation of red blood cells and is often called the 'anti-anaemic factor'. Other parts protect the nervous system, the heart and the intestines. Vitamin B is present in wheat germ, yeast and liver.

Vitamin C is found in nearly all fresh vegetables and fruits, especially in oranges, blackcurrants and fresh salads. It is destroyed by cooking or preserving. The body cannot store Vitamin C so fresh supplies are needed daily. Vitamin C promotes rapid healing of wounds and increases the body's power to ward off infection.

Vitamin D is the guardian of the bones. It is present in dairy produce, cod-liver oil and animal fats. It is also produced by the action of the rays of the sun on the skin.

Vitamin E protects the reproductive system and regulates the fat content of the blood. It is found in wheat germ oil, egg yolks and liver.

Vitamin K is essential for the clotting of the blood. It is found in liver and green vegetables.

7. ROUGHAGE

This is the name given to the indigestible parts of vegetable foods, which we need, however, to give bulk to the contents of the bowel and so prevent constipation.

Calories

A calorie is a unit of heat and is a term used to describe the energy value of food. An adult doing quiet work requires about 2,000, and a manual labourer on heavy work may require up to 4,000 calories each day. People vary a good deal between these two extremes, depending on the amount of energy they use. A child of fourteen needs about the same as an adult because of his rapid growth and use of energy. A normal diet is one which supplies an adequate number of calories to keep a person at his correct weight and enable him to do his work satisfactorily, and, in the case of a child to allow growth to take place properly.

A one-year-old child needs 44 calories a day for each pound he weighs. The diet for everyone should contain all the essential parts of food in adequate quantities.

Here are a few calorie values:

Milk	about	20	in 1 ounce (400 in 1 pint)
Butter	,,	220	,, ,, ,,
Cheese	,,	110	,, ,, ,,
Flour	,,	100	,, ,, ,,
Ice Cream	,,	60	,, ,, ,,
Potatoes	,,	25	,, ,, ,,
Bacon	,,	115	,, ,, ,,
Biscuits	,,	150	,, ,, ,,
Bread	,,	70	,, ,, ,,
Sugar	,,	120	,, ,, ,,

These are the figures we have to watch carefully—when we are watching our own figures!

All diets, whether for slimming or for fattening, in health or in disease, are built up from these calorie values.

Metabolism means all the changes which occur in the body when food is taken in and broken down, absorbed, and built up again into cells and tissues. It involves the use of oxygen which is essential for all these processes, and the giving off of carbon dioxide and water, with the continuous production of heat and energy.

Basal metabolism is the activity which continues even when the body is at rest. The basal metabolic rate (BMR) can be measured by a special apparatus, and is useful in the diagnosis of certain conditions, e.g. over-active thyroid.

27

The Digestive System

The digestive system consists of:

> *The alimentary tract,* the channel along which food passes from the mouth to the anus, and

> *The organs connected with it,* viz.:

The tongue	The pancreas
The teeth	The liver
The salivary glands	The gall-bladder

The *mouth,* the entrance to the digestive tract, is bounded by the cheeks and lips at the sides and in front, the hard palate above, and the tongue below.

The *teeth* (described with the skeletal system) form before birth, so the diet of the mother during pregnancy is an important factor in determining the quality of the baby's teeth.

Mastication of the more solid food makes the teeth sink and rise in their sockets and this has a massaging effect on the gums, promoting circulation in the pulp.

The *salivary glands* open into the mouth in front of the ear, under the tongue and under the angle of the jaw. They make saliva, which keeps the mouth moist, softens food and helps swallowing. The two glands in front of the ear are called the *parotid glands*. It is these which become inflamed in the disease called *mumps,* or they may become infected if a patient's mouth is allowed to become dirty.

The Digestive System

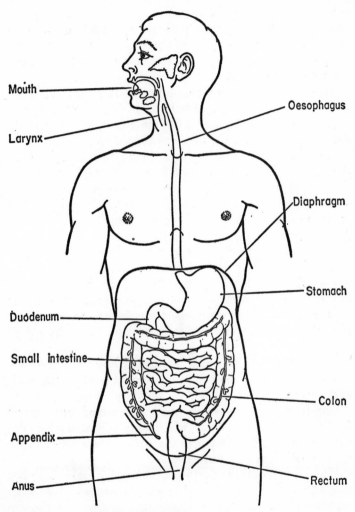

Mouth

Larynx

Oesophagus

Diaphragm

Stomach

Duodenum

Small intestine

Colon

Appendix

Anus

Rectum

FIG. 35. THE ALIMENTARY TRACT

The *pharynx* is a cone-shaped cavity at the back of the mouth. It has seven openings. They are: the larynx; those into the two Eustachian tubes, which pass up to the middle ear; the mouth; the oesophagus; the posterior openings into the cavity of the nose; and, at the back of the tongue and opening out of the pharynx, two tubes, the trachea or windpipe in front, and the oesophagus or food passage behind.

The *oesophagus* is a muscular tube 9 to 11 inches long which goes through the diaphragm and opens into the stomach.

The *stomach* is a bag shaped like the letter J. It lies below the diaphragm in front of the pancreas and spleen.

The place where the oesophagus enters the stomach is called the cardiac opening and the food passes out into the duodenum at the pyloric end. These two openings are guarded by *sphincters,* which are tight rings of muscle which open and close at intervals, so preventing the stomach from filling or emptying too quickly.

The *small intestine* is about 23 feet long, and is arranged in coils held in place by the *peritoneum,* a strong, smooth, colourless membrane, which is attached to the back of the abdominal cavity. It covers all the abdominal organs, preventing friction between them. It has many blood vessels and, for this reason, peritonitis, or inflammation of the peritoneum, is a very serious condition.

The first part of the small intestine is called the *duodenum* and secretions from the common bile duct and the pancreatic duct pass into it.

The folds of the small intestine are covered with minute finger-like projections or *villi,* which absorb digested food. The villi are so tiny that they give the wall of the small intestine the appearance of very fine velvet.

Where the small intestine joins the *large intestine* there is a worm-like structure 3 to 4 inches long, known as the *appendix.* Its value in man is not fully understood, and we only know of its presence when it becomes inflamed—appendicitis, which is cured by a simple operation.

The large intestine is divided into the caecum, the colon

and the rectum. The *caecum* is the part where the small intestine joins the large intestine. The *colon* is the part which passes up the right side, bends under the liver to pass across under the stomach, then bends downwards and curls in the shape of a letter S through the pelvis. Its last 6 to 8 inches is called the *rectum,* which is guarded by another sphincter muscle, the *anus.*

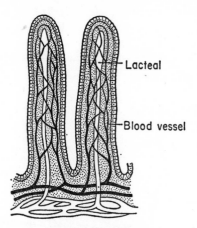

FIG. 36. THE VILLI

The *pancreas,* which lies behind the stomach, stretches from the spleen to the duodenum and is made up of grape-like clusters of cells arranged in lobes. It is 5 inches long, 2 inches wide, and weighs between 2 and 3 ounces. This gland secretes an important digestive fluid and by means of special cells known as the *islets of Langerhans* it secretes *insulin,* which helps the body to make proper use of sugar. When insulin is deficient, the disease called *diabetes* occurs.

The *liver* is the largest gland in the body and weighs about three pounds. It is situated in the upper part of the abdomen on the right side under the diaphragm.

The liver is made up of countless cells, which are surrounded by many blood vessels which come from the digestive organs.

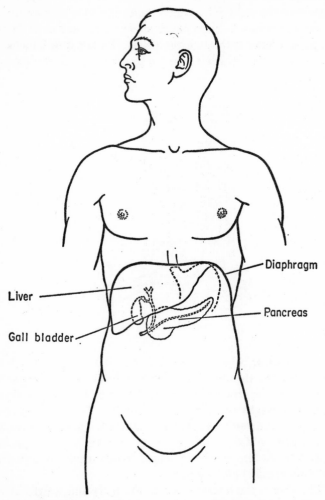

FIG. 37. THE RELATIVE POSITIONS OF THE DIAPHRAGM, THE LIVER, THE GALL BLADDER AND THE PANCREAS

The Digestive System

Functions of the Liver

1. It makes bile which helps in the digestion of fats.
2. It stores glucose in the form of glycogen until it is needed.
3. It makes some of the protective substances which the blood carries to fight bacteria.
4. It removes urea, the waste part of protein foods, and sends it to the kidneys to be excreted.
5. It makes some of the blood proteins.
6. It makes a substance, *heparin,* which prevents blood from clotting *inside* the body.

The *gall-bladder,* a pear-shaped sac on the under surface of the liver, is about 3 to 4 inches long and 1 inch wide, and is capable of holding about nine drachms of bile. It serves as a reservoir for bile in the intervals between digestion.

Digestion

Digestion is the separation of food into its simplest parts so that it can be utilized by the body.

Food is taken in at the mouth, masticated by the teeth, softened and moistened by the saliva, which is made of water, salts, and an enzyme which helps to digest cooked starches. The food is then swallowed and passed down the oesophagus into the stomach.

Now all the different muscle fibres start to work. A bit of the tube in front of the food opens up, and the bit behind closes, so that the food is pushed along and cannot go back. This happens even when you are standing on your head! This work of the muscles is called *peristalsis.*

The muscular walls of the stomach contract and roll the food from side to side, bringing it into contact with the *gastric juice.* This contains *hydrochloric acid,* which destroys germs and helps the enzymes to do their work. It takes about 3 hours for a mixed meal to be digested in the stomach.

In the duodenum food is acted upon by *bile*, and by the ferments of the pancreatic juice.

The small intestine makes enzymes which complete the digestion of sugars and starches into simple glucose, and help in the final breakdown of proteins into amino-acids.

Bile breaks down fat, has an antiseptic action on food, makes the food alkaline, and stimulates peristalsis.

Finally, in the form of amino-acids (proteins), glucose (carbohydrates), and fatty acids, the foodstuffs pass through the thin walls of the villi into the blood vessels and lymphatics.

By the time the food reaches the large intestine, 90% of its nourishment has been taken up and it remains only for water and some salts to be absorbed; then the waste matter in the form of faeces enters the last part of the colon, and produces a sensation of fullness. This feeling sends a message to the spinal cord, which in turn sends a message down a motor nerve to the anal sphincters, causing them to open and empty the rectum. In the baby this happens automatically, but as the infant grows it is able to learn to control the action. It is important that this action should be performed at a regular time every day. In this way constipation can be prevented.

DISORDERS OF THE DIGESTIVE SYSTEM

Peptic ulcer

An ulcer is an area where the skin or mucous membrane has broken down, and the tissues beneath are being slowly destroyed. When ulcers occur in the stomach or duodenum, they cause burning pain, all kinds of indigestion, and make the sufferer very unhappy and irritable.

To make sure if an ulcer is present, the doctor will ask for a series of X-ray pictures to be taken after a barium meal. Barium is a substance which outlines the digestive tract and shows up any abnormality.

The treatment is then rest, freedom from worry, a very carefully planned diet, and medicines which make the acid juice of the stomach alkaline. The two dreaded complications are *perforation,* which happens if the ulcer eats right through the walls of the organ, and *haematemesis*—severe bleeding following the same thing happening to a blood vessel. Knowing these, the nurse will watch the patient for signs of sudden collapse or the vomiting of blood. Blood passed in the stool *(melaena)* must also be reported.

Gastroenteritis

This is inflammation of the lining of stomach and intestines and is usually caused by germs taken in by food or milk. It often occurs during the summer months as an epidemic. It is especially dangerous to young children. It comes on suddenly with acute pain, vomiting, diarrhoea, sweating, shivering, the temperature and pulse rate rise, and the patient can be very ill in a few hours.

Treatment aims first at replacing the fluid lost from the body, which leads to the condition called *dehydration* (loss of water). This is always serious, whatever the cause (it occurs in burns too), because it reduces the amount of fluid available to carry vital salts and blood cells round the body. Fluid is put back by intravenous injection if the patient is very ill, or by special feeds or glucose drinks by mouth.

The other important point to be remembered is the danger of the spread of infection, especially in children's and geriatric wards. All patients suffering from diarrhoea must be barrier nursed (p. 139).

The dysenteries are types of enteritis caused by special bacteria, but the principles of treatment are the same.

Cholecystitis

Here the gall-bladder is involved. This inflammation is most commonly caused by the presence of gall-stones. The symptoms range from indigestion, especially after eating fats, to severe attacks of local pain *(colic)*. There may be *jaundice,* which is the term for a yellow colour of the skin, caused in this case by a stone blocking the bile duct so that bile cannot pass into the duodenum and goes into the blood stream instead.

This condition too can be diagnosed by a series of X-ray pictures taken after the patient has swallowed a special dye which outlines the gall-bladder.

The treatment is usually removal of the gall-bladder.

Peritonitis

Inflammation of the peritoneum used to be the most dreaded of all abdominal conditions, but today, although the patient will still be seriously ill, modern treatment ensures that he has a fine chance of recovery. Peritonitis is a complication of such things as the bursting of an appendix abscess, the perforation of an ulcer, or a direct wound.

It is treated by surgical drainage, resting the digestive tract and giving large doses of the antibiotic drug which the surgeon thinks best.

INTESTINAL OBSTRUCTION

The old-fashioned term 'stoppage' was really a good description of this dangerous condition, because the passage of everything through the bowel is stopped. It is closely associated with peritonitis. It can happen anywhere in the intestines, but is commoner in the large bowel.

The causes are:

1. *Intussusception* (this is a very long word, but if you break it up into small ones it will be easier to remember). You will only see this in babies, sometimes when they have just been weaned. It means that a small piece of ileum has been drawn into the colon, rather like the finger of a glove that has not been properly drawn out.

2. *Volvulus* occurs at the other end of life, to old people. It is a twisting of the gut—think of convolvulus, the twining plant. It can be caused by chronic constipation.

3. *Strangulated hernia.* This is where a rupture, due to a weak place in the muscle wall, has happened, and a bit of bowel has slipped in and got nipped, so cutting off the circulation to the part.

4. *Adhesions* after old operations sticking the walls of the gut together.

5. A *growth,* which has gradually got large enough to close the lumen of the bowel. (Lumen means the actual space in the middle of a tube.)

Whatever the cause, the patient quickly becomes very ill and shocked. He has acute pain, vomiting and distension and his pulse rate rises.

The treatment is operation as quickly as possible. If some of the bowel has died (gangrene), a portion will be removed and the two living ends sewn together. Sometimes an opening is made between the bowel and the outside skin to allow faeces to escape (a *colostomy*).

Afterwards, the stomach will be kept empty by suction through a tube; fluids will be given intravenously; antibiotic drugs will be injected to combat infection and careful nursing will be necessary to prevent complications. The majority of these cases make a good recovery.

28

How the Body Gets Rid of Waste: The Excretory System

When the body has burnt up its food, and taken its energy from it, it has to get rid of the waste as soon as possible. This is called *excretion*.

The chief excretory organs are the kidneys, which rid the body of the end products of protein metabolism in the urine. The lungs get rid of carbon dioxide and water in the expired air; and waste material from the digestive tract is excreted by the bowel in the faeces.

The Kidneys

The kidneys, the principal organs of excretion, are two dark red bean-shaped organs, each weighing 4 to 5 ounces and measuring about $4 \times 2\frac{1}{2} \times 1$ inch. They are embedded in fat, one on either side of the vertebral column in the lumbar region and lie behind the peritoneum.

The impurities from the blood are filtered through the kidneys into a system of collecting tubes, and turned into urine which is conveyed along the *ureters*, two ducts about the thickness of a lead pencil, to the *bladder*, a hollow muscular organ which acts as a reservoir for the urine until it is passed. The opening is guarded by another sphincter muscle.

The passing of urine, or *micturition*, normally happens when the bladder holds from six to ten ounces of urine, although an over-distended bladder may hold more than two pints. Urine dribbles continuously into the bladder from the ureters until it is

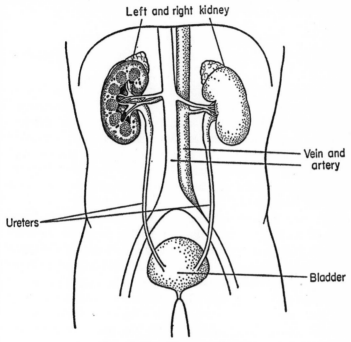

Left and right kidney

Vein and
artery

Ureters

Bladder

FIG. 38. THE URINARY SYSTEM

sufficiently full to set up a feeling of need to empty it. Control over the muscle that guards the outlet from the bladder is exerted from a centre in the brain; such control is, however, not developed in the infant and is only gradually learnt as the child grows older. Unlike the rectum, however, instead of the feeling or desire becoming dulled, the bladder will, if not emptied, become more and more distended causing acute discomfort and even pain, until control breaks down and the urine is passed.

The peritoneal coat of the bladder covers only the upper part. When the bladder is full it rises into the pelvis.

The *urethra* is a narrow passage extending from the bladder to the external urinary orifice. It is about 8 inches long in a man and $1\frac{1}{2}$ inches long in a woman.

DISORDERS OF THE URINARY TRACT

Nephritis

This applies to inflammation of any part of the kidney tissue. The kidney is a very complicated organ, and the term covers a very complicated group of conditions occurring at different ages and from different causes. Sometimes the patient recovers quickly and completely. At other times the disease goes through many stages and never really clears up. The name Bright's disease is sometimes used for it (after the name of the doctor who first described it).

The main features common to most cases are *oedema,* where parts of the body such as the feet, ankles, face, and abdomen become puffy and swollen because the fluid part of the blood drains into the tissues. *Albumin,* a blood protein, escapes in the urine, and blood is often passed as well. The patient has severe headaches and a very high blood pressure. Children may have fits, and older patients may stop making urine altogether and become unconscious, poisoned with the waste products the kidney cannot excrete *(uraemia).*

The aim of treatment in all cases is to spare the kidneys by limiting the intake of fluids, cutting down protein foods and salt in the diet, and preventing the occurrence of other infections. The nurse is responsible for keeping an accurate account of all fluids taken and passed (intake and output chart), and for testing the urine every day for albumin and blood so that the doctor can see what progress is being made.

Cystitis involves the bladder.

Infection may either be carried by the blood, or pass up from the outside, as when catheterization has been done without sterile apparatus. Both these disorders may start with rigors, a high temperature, and other signs of fever. Passing urine *(micturition)* becomes very painful and occurs very often. Blood and pus may be passed.

Rest, warmth, antibiotics, extra fluids and special medicines are given.

Renal calculus

Renal calculus means stone in the kidney. There may be one or several stones. They are usually discovered when a stone moves into the ureter and causes *renal colic*. This causes the most terrible pain. The patient rolls about in agony as the pain passes down back, thigh, and groin.

The first treatment is to relieve the pain before the victim collapses. A pain-killing drug such as morphine 16 mg. will be given. While waiting for the doctor to come, the nurse can apply heat in some form and reassure the patient that something is being done. Later, after X-rays have shown the position of the stones, they will be removed by surgery. If the kidney has been badly damaged it may have to be removed *(nephrectomy)*.

The Skin

The skin consists of an outer part, the epidermis, and an inner part, the dermis. The *epidermis* varies in thickness in different parts of the body and consists of several layers of growing epithelium which become flattened and are rubbed off and replaced by new cells underneath. Projections underneath throw it into ridges; these are particularly marked on the pads of the fingers and form a pattern which is different in every individual (fingerprints).

The epidermis has no blood vessels, nerves or glands but it contains pigment and is nourished by lymph.

The *dermis*, or true skin, lies below and is well supplied with blood vessels, lymphatic vessels, sweat glands and sebaceous or oily glands which protect the skin and prevent absorption of water. Nerve endings and hair follicles are also present.

The *nails* are horny plates on the back of the tips of the fingers and toes and are made up of flattened cells of epidermis.

The functions of the skin

1. To protect the body from invasion by germs and from injury.
2. To prevent the loss of lymph and plasma.
3. To regulate the temperature by the loss of sweat, which takes the heat from the body.
4. To excrete some waste matter, also through the sweat.
5. To give the sensation of touch, heat, cold and pain, so making us aware of what is around us.
6. To produce vitamin D, when the ultra-violet rays in sunlight fall on a fatty substance in the skin.

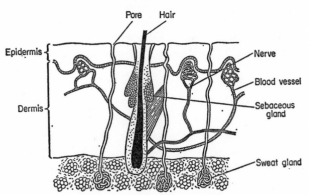

FIG. 39. SECTION OF THE SKIN

HEAT REGULATION OF THE BODY

The average normal temperature of the healthy body is from (36·1° to 37·2° C) (97° to 99° F), and varies very little whatever the surrounding atmosphere. Any upset in the balance of heat loss and heat production for more than a short period is injurious to the body cells and can be fatal, as for example in the condition known as 'heat stroke'.

The steady production of heat goes on with the normal processes of the body, i.e. taking in food, and burning it up to produce energy, movement and the activity of the glands. Some heat is absorbed from the sun and from fires. Heat is lost by radiation and conduction from the skin to the surroundings, as we all know when we leave a warm bed in the mornings, and our clothes are warm when we take them off.

Evaporation of sweat accounts for a lot of heat loss during warm weather or after violent exercise.

Some more heat is lost with breathing out.

Heat loss is helped by the dilatation of skin vessels to bring more blood to the surface to be cooled. That is why we are 'flushed' when we are hot. In cold weather the same vessels contract to keep the heat in, and we look pale.

These mechanisms are under the control of a heat-regulating centre in the brain.

Fever or pyrexia during infections is a defence on the part of the body because the high temperature makes the conditions existing in the blood and tissues unfavourable for the growth of germs.

DISORDERS OF THE SKIN

Dermatitis

This term covers a number of skin conditions, caused by irritation from substances such as disinfectants, paints, detergents, acids, etc., used in the course of work, so it is usually seen on the hands.

Eczema

Eczema is a very irritating condition which starts as redness, then tiny white blisters are seen, which discharge and run together and form crusts. Some tense, nervous children are prone to it.

Impetigo

This complaint is very infectious among children. It is caused by germs which attack the skin of poorly nourished or dirty children. It is usually seen round the mouth and nose. A child with this condition should be isolated from other children on a ward.

Psoriasis

Psoriasis shows itself as dry, scaly patches with a silvery appearance. There may be only one small patch or the whole body may be covered. The cause is unknown.

Shingles

This is a series of painful blisters along the course of a nerve. It is caused by a virus, and is most common round the chest or over one eye.

Urticaria or nettle rash

This appears as large white wheals that itch intensely. It occurs in people who are sensitive to certain foods or substances.

There is no specific treatment for any of the above. Each patient is treated individually.

Skin diseases caused by parasites are dealt with in Chapter 4.

29

The Factories of the Body: The Endocrine Glands

A *gland* is an organ which can pick materials out of the blood and can turn them into a substance which becomes the *secretion* of the gland. (A secretion is passed into the blood stream and an excretion is passed right out of the body.)

Some glands, such as the *liver, spleen, salivary glands, pancreas,* make secretions which are of use to the body. Others make fluids containing wastes, like the *kidneys* and *sweat glands*. These are considered elsewhere. Another important group have no ducts or tubes to lead their secretion out, but pour it directly into the blood stream again. These are the *endocrine glands*. Their secretions are called *hormones*.

The Endocrine Glands

1. THE PITUITARY GLAND - MASTER OF ALL GLANDS

This little gland lies in the centre of the skull, in the middle of the sphenoid bone. It produces several secretions, one of which influences the growth of bones. Under-secretion during childhood produces dwarfism or considerable undersize, while over-secretion will cause the individual to become a giant.

The pituitary exerts a controlling influence on all the other glands in the body.

It is so important that it has been named 'the leader of the endocrine orchestra'.

2. THE THYROID GLAND

This lies in the neck, just above the trachea. It controls the rate of metabolism, and so the rate of growth of the body and development of the mind. It uses iodine obtained from the food to make its secretion, *thyroxine*. Too much of this secretion causes *Graves's disease* or *exophthalmic goitre*. Too little results in a backward condition of childhood called *cretinism*. If under-secretion starts in adult life it is known as *myxoedema*.

3. THE PARATHYROIDS

These are four small bodies, two on either side of the thyroid at the back. They control the amount of calcium in the blood and in the bones. Any disturbance of their function can have serious results.

4. THE THYMUS GLAND

The thymus gland is a lymph gland situated in the chest in front of the heart. It is thought to be concerned with the development of the sex glands, holding back their functions until the proper age. About the time of puberty or early adult life it disappears.

5. THE SUPRARENAL GLANDS

These lie at the upper end of each kidney. Adrenaline produced in the central part, or medulla, of these glands is released into the blood stream in time of stress and prepares the body for 'fight or flight' by raising the blood pressure, quickening the pulse, deepening the breathing, and generally tensing the body up to meet danger, working in a very similar way to the sympathetic nervous system.

The outer part, or cortex, of the suprarenal glands produces at least three different groups of hormones; one of these is the cortisone group, which is concerned with the control of the metabolism of proteins and carbohydrates; a second group influences the retention of salt and water in the body, while a third group is concerned with the development of the secondary sex characteristics.

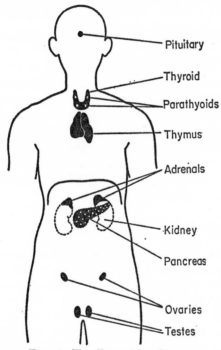

FIG. 40. THE ENDOCRINE GLANDS

6. THE ISLETS OF LANGERHANS

These are special cells found in the pancreas. They make the very important *insulin*, which controls the amount of sugar in the blood. When insulin is deficient, *diabetes mellitus* results. (See p. 256.)

7. THE OVARIES AND THE TESTES

These are the female and male organs which make secretions essential for reproduction. The ovaries make oestrogen and progesterone, which in turn control all the functions of female development and pregnancy.

The testes make testosterone, which controls normal male development.

Disorders of the Endocrine System

Addison's Disease

As we have seen, the suprarenal glands have many jobs, so if parts of them become diseased there will be some serious results. The chief feature of such diseases is great wasting and weakness which prostrates the patient so that he can no longer go on working. The blood pressure may fall so low that he collapses. Such a patient may be recognized by the peculiar bronze colour of his skin. Treatment is now by giving the hormone he lacks in the form of cortisone according to his needs.

Diabetes Mellitus

This disease occurs when the islets of Langerhans in the pancreas do not make enough insulin. This hormone is essential for the proper use of sugar. When it is lacking, instead of sugar being turned into energy, it is simply passed out in the urine.

The onset is gradual, with loss of weight and thirst, or perhaps repeated boils or carbuncles. The disease is often only discovered when the urine is tested during an investigation. If not treated the condition will get worse until the patient may pass into the unconscious state called *diabetic coma.*

The routine treatment of diabetes is the giving of insulin by mouth or by injection, together with a controlled diet until a balance is reached and very little sugar is passed in the urine. The nurse's responsibility is to see that the dosages are given correctly and punctually.

Later, the patient will be taught enough about diabetes to enable him to act sensibly, to test his own urine and give his own injections, and to recognize when anything needs his doctor's advice. He will be told what he can eat, and how much. He should be encouraged to join the Diabetic Association which exists to help diabetics in many different ways.

Graves's Disease

This disorder of the thyroid gland is rather trying for the pupil nurse, as she may also hear it called *thyrotoxicosis, exophthalmic goitre,* or even *hyperthyroidism* as well! All these names mean that the gland is overactive. If it is swollen as well this is a *goitre.* As the secretion of the gland, thyroxine, controls metabolism, it follows that too much will cause a speed up of every function, the heart beat will be very rapid *(tachycardia)*, causing the pulse to race. There will be loss of weight because the patient burns up his food too rapidly—yet he will still be hungry. He will feel hot and sweat freely. He may have diarrhoea. He may look and feel jumpy, frightened, and may both laugh and cry for nothing. The eyes may protrude.

Treatment is medical at first, keeping the patient quiet and rested. When his general condition is better it is usual to operate and remove a good deal of the gland. The condition occurs in both sexes, but seems to be commoner in women.

30

How Life is Continued:
The Reproductive System

The reproductive system naturally differs greatly in the two sexes.

The Male Reproductive Organs

In the male the generative organs consist of an external organ, the *penis*, down the centre of which runs the *urethra*, and a system of internal glands and tubes which are concerned with the production of male cells or spermatozoa.

The testes are two oval glands which develop in the abdomen shortly before birth and descend along the inguinal canal to the *scrotum*, which is a pouch-like structure outside the body. Each testis consists of a mass of special coiled tubules and produces the important secretion testosterone and male cells or spermatozoa.

The seminal vesicle is connected to the seminal duct and acts as a reservoir for the seminal fluid.

The prostate gland, which surrounds the orifice of the urethra as it leaves the bladder, is about the size of a chestnut. It is thought to secrete another fluid essential for reproduction.

The Female Reproductive Organs

In the female the generative organs consist of:

The uterus
The uterine (Fallopian) tubes
The ovaries
The vagina

These organs are all internal. The external genitals are collectively called the vulva.

The *uterus* is a hollow, muscular, pear-shaped organ situated behind the bladder and in front of the rectum. It has a very strong muscular coat and is held in position by strong ligaments.

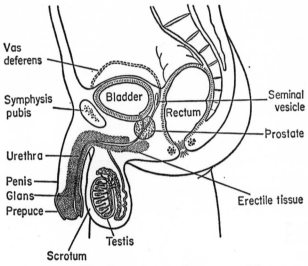

FIG. 41. THE REPRODUCTIVE ORGANS IN A MAN

Normally it is 3×2 inches in size, but in pregnancy it reaches 12×10 inches. It is this organ which contains and nourishes the infant until birth.

Connecting the uterus with the vagina is the *cervix*, or neck, and from the widest part of the body of the uterus, the two *Fallopian tubes* are given off. They collect the ova from the ovaries and pass them into the uterus.

The *ovaries*. Every month after puberty the ovaries produce ova which are swept along into the uterus by the Fallopian tubes. Fertilization means that an ovum or egg cell has united with a male cell, or spermatozoa, usually in a Fallopian tube. If all goes well this now double cell should fix itself on to the uterine wall from which it will draw its nourishment, going through many stages for 36 weeks until it becomes a full term infant ready for birth.

When fertilization does not take place, the monthly feature known as *menstruation* occurs. This simply means that the ovum, along with the mucous membrane lining of the uterus, and some of the superficial blood supply, is discarded and passed out. After this the uterus rapidly repairs itself and again prepares for the reception of the next ovum.

The *vagina* is the passage leading from the outside of the body to the cervix of the uterus. It curves upwards and backwards. Its lining is puckered to allow for great distension during childbirth.

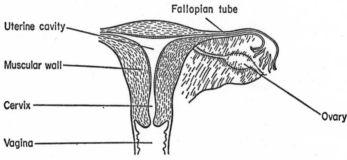

FIG. 42. THE REPRODUCTIVE ORGANS IN A WOMAN

The *external organs,* or *vulva,* include the orifice of the urethra, through which the urine is excreted, and the orifice of the vagina, which allows the fully developed infant to escape from the uterus.

The *perineum* is the expanse of skin between the vaginal orifice and the anus. It is an area very liable to injury during the process of childbirth.

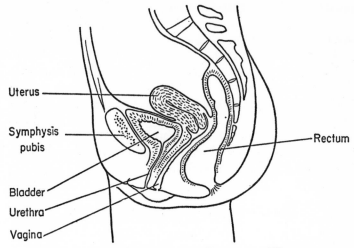

FIG. 43. SECTION THROUGH THE PELVIS OF A WOMAN

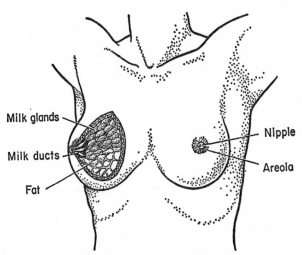

FIG. 44. THE BREAST, SHOWING MILK GLANDS

261

Puberty is the period at which the generative organs become capable of fulfilling their functions.

The menopause is the period at which the reproductive organs cease to function although it is possible to conceive up to two years after the last period.

The breasts contain the milk glands. These glands increase in size at puberty, and the cells lining the milk ducts become active when pregnancy occurs and secrete the milk, which is specially adapted to the requirements of the normal infant and moreover contains antitoxins and antibacteriological substances which have been formed in the mother's blood and which protect the infant from infection.

Disorders of the Reproductive System

MALE

Prostate gland enlargement

This is a common disorder of older men. The gland tends to get bigger as life advances, and sometimes it presses on the back of the urethra and stops the urine from flowing properly, so that some always remains in the bladder. This may become infected, making the patient feel ill. It may even cause pressure upwards so that the kidneys are hindered in their work and the waste products are kept in the blood *(uraemia)*.

The usual treatment is first to drain the bladder by an artificial opening (suprapubic drainage) and, when the patient is well enough, to remove the gland.

FEMALE

The disorders of the female reproductive system form a special branch of medicine called *gynaecology*. The nurse will learn about them when she works in a gynaecological ward. Meanwhile, she may find it useful to know a few terms, e.g. those given on the next page.

Fibroids

Benign (that is, not cancer) tumours in the womb or uterus. They are fairly common, and are best removed before they cause trouble by pressing on other organs, or interfere with pregnancy.

Leucorrhoea

Leucorrhoea means a white discharge from the vagina. A small amount is normal, but if it becomes yellow or frothy it must be investigated. It may be caused by a tiny creature called *Trichomonas.*

Dysmenorrhoea

Dysmenorrhoea means painful periods. There are many different causes and if it is severe the sufferer should get advice and follow out the doctor's instructions. It is often cured by a simple operation called *dilatation* and *curettage.* This opens up the channel along which the blood must pass, so enabling it to flow more freely, and at the same time the doctor is able to see if there is any deeper trouble.

31

How We Recognize Our World:
The Special Senses

The special senses are five in number. They are sight, hearing, smell, taste, and touch.

The Organ of Sight

This consists of:

> The eyeball
> The optic nerve
> The centre for vision in the brain
> The conjunctiva
> The lacrimal, or tear-making, apparatus
> The muscles which move the eyeballs
> The eyelids
> The eyebrows

The eyeball is covered with conjunctiva, a thin transparent membrane, which is folded back over the surfaces of the upper and lower lids. It is moved by six muscles arranged so as to move the eyeball up and down and from side to side, as well as obliquely.

The coloured part of the eye is called the *iris*. In the centre of the iris is a hole, the *pupil*, which allows light to enter the eye. Behind the pupil is the *lens* which focuses the light on the back

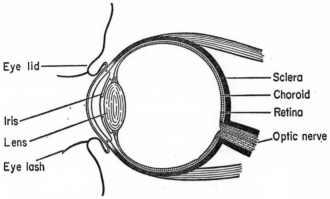

Eye lid

Iris

Lens

Eye lash

Sclera

Choroid

Retina

Optic nerve

FIG. 45. VERTICAL SECTION OF THE EYE

of the eye where the *optic nerve* lies. The optic nerve transmits the image to the brain and we become conscious of the object at which we are looking.

Abnormal vision occurs when the rays do not meet exactly at

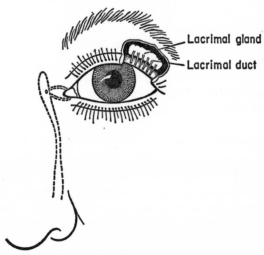

Lacrimal gland

Lacrimal duct

FIG. 46. THE TEAR APPARATUS

265

this point, because the eyeball is too long or too short, and needs to be corrected by the wearing of glasses.

Tears, which keep the eye moist and serve to remove foreign bodies, are secreted by the lacrimal glands and pass from the outer to the inner side of the eye through the lacrimal ducts into the nose, any excess flowing down the cheek.

The eyebrows prevent perspiration from entering the eye.

The eyelids protect the eye and by their blinking movement keep the front of the eye free from dust and help to move tears across the conjunctival sac.

DISORDERS OF THE EYE

Cataract

The lens, which is normally clear like glass to let the light rays through, becomes cloudy or opaque, so that the patient sees less and less. The lens can, however, be removed by operation, and its place is taken by artificial lens in spectacles.

Conjunctivitis is inflammation of the delicate membrane covering the front of the eye. It is treated with hot bathing and the instillation of eyedrops which will be ordered by the doctor.

Glaucoma

The eyeball is filled with a watery fluid which should always remain the same in amount and pressure. In glaucoma these increase, there will be great pain, and in time the pressure on the retina would cause blindness.

This condition too is treated by operation.

Ophthalmia neonatorum

This is an eye infection of the newborn baby, caused by pus entering the eye during birth. Silver nitrate drops are instilled at birth in all cases to prevent this condition developing; if it does occur the eyes look red and sore and discharge pus. They must be treated quickly with large doses of penicillin or the child may go blind. The cause is usually the germ of one of the venereal diseases, gonorrhoea.

How We Recognize Our World: the Special Senses

The Organ of Hearing

This consists of:

The external ear
The middle ear
The internal ear
The auditory nerve
The centre for hearing in the brain

The *external ear* consists of the outside part which we see when we look at someone and the ear passage leading to the interior.

Stretched across the end of the ear passage is the *ear drum*, separating the external ear from the *middle ear*.

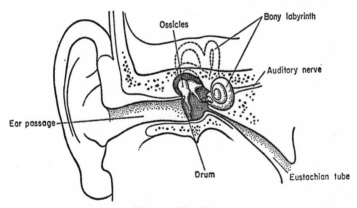

FIG. 47. THE EAR

The middle ear contains three tiny levers of bone called the *ossicles* and the *inner ear* consists of a *bony labyrinth* filled with fluid. Attached to the bony labyrinth are the fibres of the *auditory nerve*.

Sound waves pass along the ear passage causing the drum to vibrate. The vibration sets the ossicles in motion and so transmits the sound waves to the bony labyrinth. Signals from

267

the bony labyrinth are carried by the auditory nerve to the brain where they are interpreted as the sounds we hear.

The *Eustachian tube* connects the middle ear to the nasal cavity and serves to balance the pressure between the middle ear and the outside air. When we swallow the Eustachian tube opens and this prevents discomfort or injury to the drum when the air pressure is changing quickly—for example, at take-off in an aircraft.

DISORDERS OF THE EAR

Otitis media

Inflammation of the middle ear. It is commonest in childhood, and causes painful earache. Infection spreads up the Eustachian tube from a sore throat or during measles or scarlet fever.

Mastoiditis

Mastoiditis may be the next stage, when the tiny air spaces in the mastoid process of the temporal bone are infected. As it is so near the brain it would be dangerous if left, so the bone has to be opened and drained. Antibiotic drugs help to clear up both these conditions quickly.

The Organ of Smell

This is contained in the nerve endings of the *olfactory nerve* which pass through tiny holes in the ethmoid bone, to be distributed over the mucous membrane of the upper part of the nose. The impulses are conveyed to a special centre in the brain.

Substances capable of being smelled, must be dissolved in the form of gases. This explains why sniffing enables us to smell better. It brings the gas nearer to the nerve endings. The sense of smell is very quickly fatigued, and for this reason it is very important to pay attention to a disagreeable odour at once lest one should cease to notice it.

The Sense of Taste

This lies in the tongue, in taste buds situated mostly at the sides and base of the tongue. These contain special cells with nerve endings from the cranial nerve of taste. Substances cannot be tasted, however, until they are dissolved in the watery secretion of the mouth and the salivary glands.

Salty tastes are perceived most easily all over the tongue, but the sides of the tongue are most sensitive to acids and the back to bitter substances.

The Sense of Touch

The nerves of the skin transmit the sensations of:

Pain	Cold
Heat	Pressure or touch

Pain, although we do not like it, is essential for our wellbeing, as it enables us to know if we are being injured or leads us to investigate its cause, and so helps in the detection of disease. Often too, by compelling rest, it assists the process of healing.

All sensations felt by the skin are received by special little nerve endings which send their messages up to the brain, which tells us what we have felt.

32

How the Body is Controlled:
The Nervous System

The nervous system is the great controlling and coordinating system of the body. It is made up of the *brain*, which sends out and receives messages from all parts of the body and translates them into thought and feeling; the *spinal cord*, along which these messages are relayed, and the *nerves*, which carry the messages.

Motor nerves carry messages from the brain and cord to the muscles, causing movement of some kind.

Sensory nerves carry sensations to the brain. These include those of sight, hearing, smell, taste, pain, heat, cold, sense of position.

The Central Nervous System

The central nervous system controls the voluntary muscles of the body and limbs and consists of the brain and spinal cord, twelve pairs of *cranial nerves* coming from the brain, and thirty-one pairs of *spinal nerves*.

THE BRAIN

The *brain* is situated in the cranium and is covered by three coverings called *meninges*. It consists of nerve cells, or grey matter, and nerve fibres, or white matter, on the inside.

The chief parts of the brain are:

1. *The cerebrum, or great brain.* This is divided in half by a deep groove running from front to back. Its surface is thrown into folds called *convolutions*, and fissures divide it into lobes.

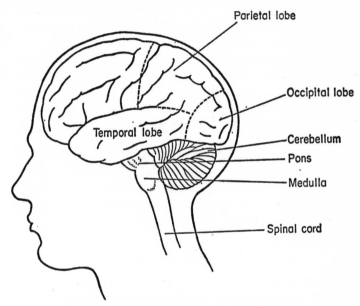

Parietal lobe

Occipital lobe

Temporal lobe

Cerebellum

Pons

Medulla

Spinal cord

FIG. 48. THE CHIEF PARTS OF THE BRAIN

Every lobe has a different function. The halves, or hemispheres, contain *ventricles,* spaces which contain *cerebrospinal fluid,* which acts as a water cushion for the brain and cord. Sometimes, in fractures of the base of the skull, this fluid may escape from the ears.

The function of the cerebrum is to control the movements of all the muscles of the head, limbs and trunk. It is the seat of the intellect, of memory, reason, thought and the emotions.

It is by its means that we appreciate all sensations, pleasant or painful.

It also contains the motor centres which send out messages to the muscles, telling them what movements to perform to carry out all our actions.

2. *The cerebellum, or little brain.* This lies below the cerebrum. It is only about the size of a small orange. Its function is to control the balance of the body and make the muscles work together smoothly.

3. *The pons Varolii.* This is a bridge of fibres, which joins together all the parts of the brain.

4. *The medulla oblongata.* This lies at the back, and is continuous with the spinal cord. Although in a humble position, possibly for its protection, it is of supreme importance, because it contains the vital centres of life which preserves the functions of the heart and circulation, of breathing, swallowing and vomiting.

Twelve pairs of cranial nerves emerge from the brain. They are both sensory and motor, and include the *optic* nerve of sight, the *auditory* nerve of hearing, and the great *vagus* nerve, which runs far down into the body to supply all the internal organs, and the nerves of taste and smell.

THE SPINAL CORD

The spinal cord is about 18 inches long. It passes out of the skull through a hole in the occipital bone and is contained in the canal made by the arches of the vertebrae.

At regular intervals the spinal cord gives off thirty-one pairs of nerves, which conduct impulses from the brain to all parts of the body, and back again to the brain.

An impulse, starting from one side of the brain, passes through a cell in the spinal cord to a nerve on the opposite side and so to a muscle.

In the cervical (neck) and lumbar (loin) regions important networks of nerves are given off which supply the arm, the hand, the leg and the foot.

If a person wishes to move his right hand, the part of the brain controlling the right hand informs the exchange in the spinal cord and a message is sent along another nerve to the muscles of the right hand, and so it is moved.

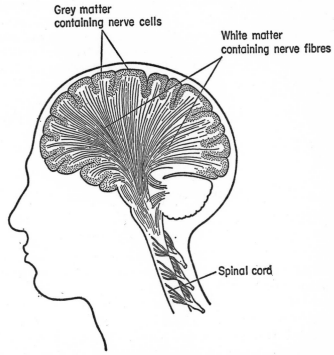

FIG. 49. DIAGRAM OF NERVE FIBRES LEADING FROM THE NERVE CELLS TO THE SPINAL CORD

Reflex actions are those which are automatic, e.g. removing the hand suddenly from a hot surface or a pin prick; closing the eye when the dust enters. These actions are controlled through centres in the spinal cord without reference to higher centres in the brain.

A conditioned reflex is a trained one, like training a child to pass urine in the proper place, or to open the bowels at a regular time. This leaves the brain free to think, reason, and carry out those actions which require *conscious* thought.

The Autonomic Nervous System

This part of the nervous system controls those organs which are not under the control of the will. Breathing, bowel movement, the making and secreting of digestive juices and hormones, blood pressure, and childbirth are some of the functions looked after in this manner. This serves to relieve the busy conscious brain of having to concentrate on the details of existence every second of the day and night. The autonomic centres are rather like Local Government offices, which, though under the control of Parliament, do not have to bother the central Government with every small detail of daily life in their areas.

Disorders of the Nervous System

Cerebral palsy

This condition is one which every nurse will have heard of but which she may not see unless she works in a special Home or a child suffering from it is admitted for some other illness. It is a condition present at birth, caused by damage to the brain cells which control the muscles. Instead of learning to make normal, graceful movements, such a child has no control over his limbs. He cannot walk, dress or feed himself. He may dribble, and cannot speak intelligibly. The limbs are stiff and ungainly, so these children are also called 'spastics'.

These cases used to be considered hopeless imbeciles, but we know now that, hidden behind these terrible disabilities, their intelligence is often normal or even higher, and with devoted care and training they can be made, in many cases, into happy and useful people.

Disseminated or multiple sclerosis

This is a fairly common disease in which small areas of nerve

274

tissue become abnormal and cease to carry messages properly from the brain to the body. These areas are scattered all through the brain and spinal cord, so different symptoms appear as different nerves are affected. They range from loss of feeling in a limb to loss of sight in one eye. Gradually more and more symptoms appear until in the end the patient becomes paralysed and helpless.

Treatment aims at keeping the patient going as long as possible, and treating each trouble as it appears.

Epilepsy

The cause of this is not known. Some disturbance of the brain causes the epileptic to fall down in a fit which always goes through three stages, the first where he is stiff, eyes staring and teeth clenched, followed by violent convulsions in which he may bite his tongue or otherwise hurt himself. This stage is followed by deep sleep or confusion.

The treatment is by drugs which have to be taken all through life to reduce the fits, and if one does occur, to prevent any injury happening to the patient.

Meningitis

In this condition the covering of the brain becomes inflamed. It is always caused by bacteria. The patient, usually a child, complains of severe headache. He turns his head away from the light, and his back becomes stiff and his neck arched backwards. There is a high temperature and the patient is very ill. The doctor will soon do a *lumbar puncture* to get a specimen of the fluid from the spinal canal, and as soon as he knows what germ is present large doses of the right antibiotic drug will be given, some by intra-muscular injection and some straight into the spinal canal.

The nurse will do all her part of feeding and washing the patient with tenderness, knowing that she is handling a very sick child who is in great pain.

Poliomyelitis (infantile paralysis)

This is an infectious fever caused by a virus which can destroy some of the motor nerve cells in the spinal cord, so that the part which they serve becomes paralysed. Paralysis can range from slight weakness to involvement of almost the whole body. The illness starts with the same symptoms as most fevers—headache, vomiting, a high temperature, but paralysis comes on very quickly. It may be only of one leg, but in some cases the muscles used in breathing are affected, and then the patient's life is in danger unless continuous artificial respiration can be given. This is done by using a respirator.

Some patients, with good nursing, special exercises and all kinds of physiotherapy go a long way towards complete recovery. Others may not be so fortunate and are left with a permanent disability.

One of the nurse's most important jobs is to encourage and reassure and keep hope alive.

One of the most wonderful advances in modern medicine is the production of the Salk Vaccine which can now protect us all from this terrible disease. Immunization is now available for everybody, and all nurses are given this protection.

Stroke (apoplexy)

One of the commonest conditions to be nursed among the older patients in our wards is caused by the bursting of a small blood vessel in the brain, or the blocking of one by an embolism. This causes sudden loss of consciousness and paralysis of one side of the body *(hemiplegia)*. While the patient is unconscious very good nursing is essential to prevent him from choking, and to keep him free of pressure sores and retention of urine in the bladder. In fact, there is not much medical treatment possible, and everything depends on the nursing staff and physiotherapists at first, and later the occupational therapist, to get the patient on his feet again.

When he begins to recover consciousness, it may be found that he cannot speak properly. Nurses should remember that it is a very frightening thing to know what is going on and yet be unable to ask questions or ask for what one wants. It is very comforting if the nurse realizes this and talks to the patient as if he were normal, and tries to make him feel that he is safe and not cut off from human contact.

SECTION FOUR

First Aid and Bandaging

33

The Principles of First Aid

Eight thousand people die every year from accidents in their homes, quite apart from those dying on the roads. Add to this the number of those who have been seriously injured or disabled, think of the fear, grief, shock and misery of those who have lost someone dear in this way, and you will realize how important it is for EVERYONE to have some knowledge that may save life, and especially so for nurses, to whom the public will turn for help, particularly if they are in uniform.

The two chief aims of the First Aider are to save life and to prevent further injury. She must possess some knowledge, the ability to keep calm and to reassure others, and plenty of common sense.

In order to save life and prevent further injury the first aider should:

1. Check that the patient is breathing.
2. Stop any bleeding.
3. Treat for shock.
4. Cover wounds or burns.
5. Immobilize fractures.
6. Get the patient to hospital with all possible speed.

Breathing

Look at the patient's chest and see if it is moving. If not, put your head down to his nose and mouth and listen. If he is not breathing clear his airway and start mouth to mouth breathing.

Clearing his airway

1. Take out any dentures.
2. Wrap a handkerchief round your finger. Turn his head

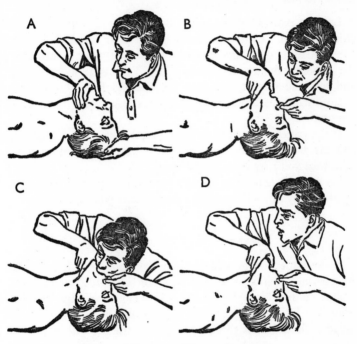

FIG. 50. MOUTH TO MOUTH BREATHING

to one side and run your finger round inside his mouth and throat to remove vomit, blood, food, water or anything else which may be stopping him from breathing.

3. Bend his head right back as far as it will go. At the same time bring his lower jaw up until his teeth are firmly closed and hold it there.

When a person stops breathing he loses consciousness. When he becomes unconscious his tongue, which is attached to his lower jaw, often falls slackly backwards, blocking his throat and making it impossible for him to breathe. With his head bent fully back and his jaws closed so that his teeth are meeting this cannot happen.

Mouth to mouth breathing

Lay the patient on his back. Bend his head *fully* back and close his jaws. Close his nostrils with your fingers. Take a deep breath and making an airtight seal with your mouth over the patient's mouth, blow into him. Take your mouth away and look sideways to see that his chest is falling as the air escapes from his lungs. Repeat this process about 12 times a minute.

If the patient is a child fit your mouth over both his mouth and his nose, and be very gentle as you breathe into him, otherwise you may damage his lungs.

Go on with mouth to mouth breathing until the patient is breathing by himself, or until a doctor tells you to stop.

BREATHING BUT UNCONSCIOUS

If the patient is breathing but unconscious put him in the semi-prone position with his head on one side, so that his tongue cannot block his airway. If possible arrange that his head is a little lower than his feet so that if he vomits, or if blood collects in his throat, the downward tilt will help it to

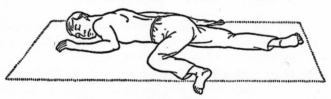

FIG. 51. THE SEMI-PRONE POSITION

drain out of his mouth instead of being breathed into his lungs, and choking him.

Never give a pillow to an unconscious patient.

If he has dentures take them out, wrap them in a handkerchief and put them in his pocket.

Bleeding

1. Raise the part, e.g. if the hand is bleeding raise the arm. This should slow or stop the bleeding. Then put on a clean dressing (a folded handkerchief would do as a pad) and bandage firmly in place.

2. If bleeding continues *do not* remove the bandage because this will disturb the clot which is forming.

Put another pad on top of it and apply another bandage more firmly, or put your hand on the bleeding point and press *hard*.

Shock

Shock is a strange condition in which all the tiny blood vessels —capillaries—get wider (dilate), so that the blood flows sluggishly through them, and it takes too long for oxygen to reach the vital centres of the brain. Think of the difference between water flowing in a wide, shallow river where it hardly seems to move, and that running in a narrow stream where it rushes along. No one knows exactly why this happens, but we do know that the main things which cause shock are:

1. Fear
2. Pain
3. Haemorrhage
4. Exposure to cold

The signs and symptoms of shock are:

skin—pale and clammy
pulse—weak and rapid
breathing—shallow and quiet

TREATMENT OF SHOCK

1. Keep the patient quiet and undisturbed. Reassure him and answer any anxious questions quietly and cheerfully.

2. If possible keep the head lower than the body, so that blood is not taken from the vital centres in the brain.

3. Prevent chilling by placing a light covering over his body, but *do not* use hot water bottles or let the patient get hot enough to sweat, or he will lose fluid from his skin and make his condition worse.

4. Give nothing by mouth at all. If an injury is found which requires surgery and an anaesthetic, there may be serious delay when it is found that the stomach is full of fluid. Transport to hospital is very quick and fluids can be given there if the Casualty Officer decides it is safe to do so.

Burns and Scalds

A *burn* is caused by *dry* heat or by chemicals.

A *scald* is caused by *moist* heat (steam) or by hot liquids.

The effects of a burn depend upon its situation and on the extent of the body surface involved.

Burns are more dangerous on the head than on the limbs. There are two degrees of burns:

1. *Superficial*. Some of the skin is destroyed, but there are patches left from which cells can spread to make new skin.
2. *Deep*. Here the skin is completely destroyed over the whole area.

All burns cause a great deal of shock, and if more than a third of the body surface is burnt, the victim is not likely to live.

FIRST AID TREATMENT FOR BURNS AND SCALDS

If the clothing is on fire pull the burning person to the ground and smother the flames with a rug, curtains or any material that is large enough.

Send for the doctor.

If possible hold the burnt area under a cold water tap, or pour cold water over it, for ten minutes. This will lessen the pain and therefore help to reduce the shock.

The burnt person is not only in great pain, he is very, very frightened. Fire is a terrifying thing. This combination of pain and fear causes profound shock, out of all proportion to the area burnt.

If the skin is destroyed over an area larger than a penny get the patient to hospital immediately. Speed is essential to save his life.

Do *not* pull off clothes which have stuck to the burn.

Do *not* prick blisters.

Cover the burns either with clean dry dressings or wrap the patient in a clean sheet.

A scalded child should be wrapped completely in a clean sheet and then in a blanket, and taken immediately to the nearest hospital. Delay in treating the severe shock may be fatal and every moment counts.

Fractures

A fracture or break in a bone may be due to violence, to disease, or to old age when the bones become brittle and snap easily.

Fractures may be:

1. *Closed*, when there is no open wound.

2. *Open* when there *is* a wound communicating with the fracture.

Signs and symptoms of a fracture

1. Pain
2. Loss of the power of movement
3. Swelling
4. Unnatural shape or position of the limb, or body
5. Shock

FIRST AID TREATMENT FOR FRACTURES

Send at once for the doctor.

Stop any bleeding and cover up any broken skin with a clean dressing or with the cleanest material available.

Reassure the patient and if possible do not move him until the doctor arrives.

If obliged to handle the part, use extreme care so as to avoid causing further injury.

It is better to tie a broken arm to the body, or a broken leg to the good leg with wide bandages, than to use makeshift splints.

Never do more than is necessary.

Fracture of the spine

Do not move the patient until it is absolutely essential. When he *must* be moved, keep him *in the position in which he was found*. If he lies curled up he must be moved curled up. If he is on his face, do not turn him. Do not try to make him more comfortable by placing a cushion under his head; if his neck is broken this may kill him. Gently work a rug under him and use this to move him. Put something soft between his legs and strap thighs, knees and ankles together.

Four people *at least* must be found to move him—more if possible.

An injured motor cyclist recently walked out of hospital completely well. He had been found lying almost in a circle. He owes his life to the ambulance men who got him to hospital without changing his position by an inch. On the other hand a woman, who had a simple fracture of one of the cervical bones, died because a well-meaning onlooker slipped a cushion under her head.

Fracture of the clavicle

Put a pad in the axilla of the injured side (a tennis ball would do). Bandage the tip of the elbow to the chest after gently putting the arm in a sling.

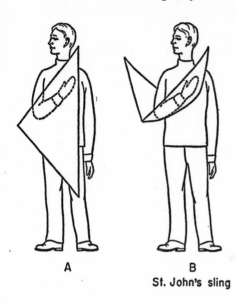
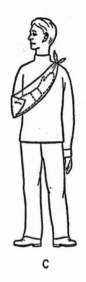

A   B   C

St. John's sling

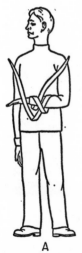
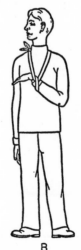

A   B

Collar and cuff

FIG. 52 TYPES OF SLING

Fracture of the humerus

Supporting the upper arm, bend the elbow. Put a narrow sling round the wrist. The weight of the arm acts as an extension. Then bind elbow to side to prevent any movement.

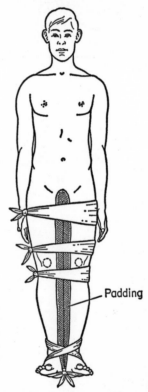

Padding

FIG. 53. SPLINTS AND BANDAGES FOR A FRACTURED FEMUR

Fracture of the pelvis

Keep the patient lying flat on his back, with a support under his knees. If he wants to pass urine try to restrain him until he reaches hospital, where a catheter will be passed by a doctor.

288

Fracture of the femur

Using as many scarves or other suitable pieces of material as necessary, tie ankles together, then legs below and above the knee, and a wide one right round both hips. Avoid pressure on the site of the break itself.

Fracture of the ribs

Place two very broad bandages round the chest, overlapping at the site of the injury to give extra support. Tell the patient to breathe out, then tie firmly on the good side. Keep the patient sitting up.

Dressings and Bandages

Most first aid kits will contain sterile dressings, roller bandages, adhesive tape and triangular bandages.

If these are not available use dry clean material for dressings, e.g. clean handkerchiefs. A scarf or tea towel can be used in place of a triangular bandage.

The purpose of a dressing is:
1. To prevent blood escaping.
2. To stop germs from getting in.

The purpose of a bandage is:
1. To keep dressings in position.
2. To give steady support to injured parts.
3. To stop bleeding by pressure.
4. To prevent movement.

Rules for bandaging

1. Place the limb in the position it will occupy when bandaged.
2. Two surfaces of skin should not be in contact. Absorbent wool or some soft material should be placed between them.

3. Secure the bandage by a couple of oblique turns round the limb.

4. Bandage from below upwards, and from within outwards. Each turn should overlap two-thirds of the preceding turn.

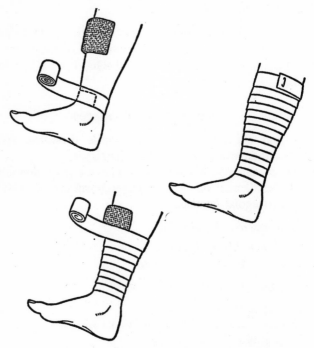

FIG. 54. APPLICATION OF ROLLER BANDAGE TO THE LEG

5. Do not apply to a limb so tightly as to cause the tips of the fingers or toes to become discoloured.

6. Do not bandage too loosely. It is of no use and is uncomfortable for the patient.

7. Never apply a damp bandage. It will shrink and become too tight.

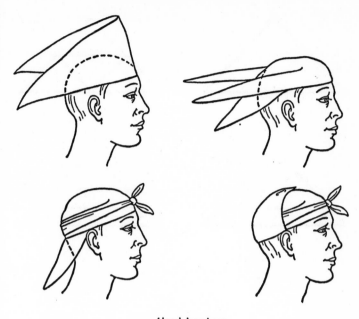

Head bandage

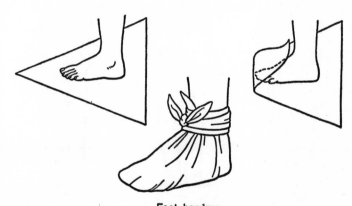

Foot bandage

FIG. 55. THE USE OF TRIANGULAR BANDAGES

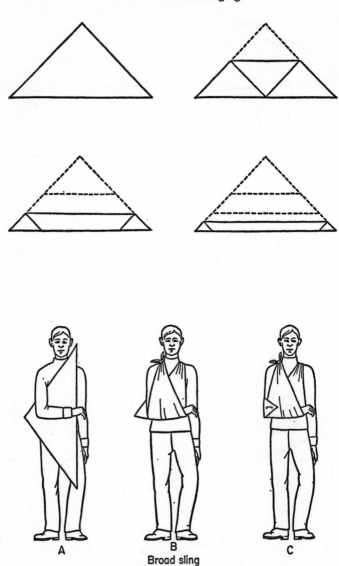

Broad sling

FIG. 56. THE USE OF TRIANGULAR BANDAGES

Triangular bandages

The first aid triangular bandage can be used as a narrow or wide bandage, or as a sling.

Miscellaneous Catastrophes

Choking

If the patient is a child hold him upside down and slap him between the shoulders.

If he is an adult get him to sit bent forward in a chair and hit him hard between the shoulders. If this does not remove the obstruction send for the doctor.

Electric shock

Switch off the current if this is possible.

If it is not possible, as on a railway line, stand on a *non-conductor*, i.e. a substance through which electricity cannot easily pass, such as a waterproof rubber sheet, matting, cork, brick, hay, bundles of newspaper or books, or wear rubber boots.

Push the victim away with a long pole.

Never stand on *metal* or on anything *damp* because moisture conducts electricity.

Use only one hand and protect it by means of rubber, dry newspaper, a felt hat or a woollen garment.

Immediately the patient is rescued apply mouth to mouth breathing. This applies also to people who have been struck by lightning. Look for and treat any burns.

Drowning

Clean any mud or seaweed from the throat with the fore-finger protected by a handkerchief. Remove dentures.

Turn the patient on his back and start mouth to mouth breathing. Continue for at least an hour or until he is breathing normally.

When he is breathing again put him in the semi-prone position with his head lower than his feet if possible.

Get him to hospital and be ready to start mouth to mouth breathing again at any time if his own breathing falters.

Heatstroke or sunstroke

Heatstroke occurs when a person has been in a situation in which he could not lose any body heat to the atmosphere from his skin in the normal way. It sometimes affects soldiers and cadets who are on training marches in full uniform, where most of the body is covered. The victim suddenly falls unconscious to the ground.

Pull him into the shade. Strip off all clothing. Pour cold water over his body and put ice on his head. If this is not available, fan him with a newspaper. When he comes round give him plenty of cold drinks.

Gas poisoning

Throw open the windows, turn off the gas, then drag the patient into the open air. Loosen tight clothing and start mouth to mouth breathing until the doctor arrives.

Hanging

Cut the patient down, supporting his body while doing so. Lay him flat and get someone to send for the doctor and the police. In the meantime start mouth to mouth breathing.

Fainting

This may be due to hunger, exhaustion or emotional causes.

Take the patient into the open air. Get him to sit down and put his head between his knees. Offer him a cup of hot, sweet tea or coffee, and some sympathy and reassurance.

Dog bite

The wound should be washed with warm water and the

patient taken to the doctor so that the injury can be inspected and, if necessary, the patient inoculated.

Poisoning

If the patient is unconscious put him in the semi-prone position and get him to hospital immediately, together with anything which may give an indication of the poison taken, e.g. pills, bottles, vomit.

If the patient is conscious look at his lips, mouth and tongue.

If they are burnt or stained give him water, milk or raw eggs to dilute the poison, and send him immediately to hospital. *Never* give him an emetic.

If they are not burnt give him an emetic, such as a tablespoon-ful of salt or mustard in a glass of water, to make him vomit as soon as possible. After he has vomited follow on with milk, water or raw egg. Get him to hospital at once.

Save all vomit and urine. Put away in a safe place any bottle, glass or cup which may have contained the poison, also any letters, telegrams or messages found on or near the patient, as soon as possible after treating him.

Nose-bleed

Get the patient to sit up with his head forward. Tell him to pinch his nostrils and stay like this for fifteen minutes. If after this time his nose is still bleeding take him to hospital.

34

Bandages and Splints in Hospital

Tubegauz bandaging

This is the form of bandaging now used in many hospitals and the nurse, with a little practice, should soon be able to use it quickly and efficiently. Tubegauz is a woven cotton bandage prepared in circular form which is applied by means of a series of metal applicators of various sizes for all parts of the body. These hold lengths of circular gauze which are cut off to the size required after the applicator has been passed several times over the area to be covered.

Crepe bandages, conforming bandages and open weave gauze bandages are also used.

Splints may be straight or moulded to the shape of the injured part. Most commonly used now are light, pliable splints made of Perspex or other plastic.

Splints can also be moulded in plaster of Paris.

Preparation for the application of plaster of Paris

Required:

Mackintosh apron ⎫
Gown   ⎬ for the surgeon
Rubber gloves   ⎪
Cotton leggings or gum boots ⎭
Mackintoshes to protect the bed and the floor

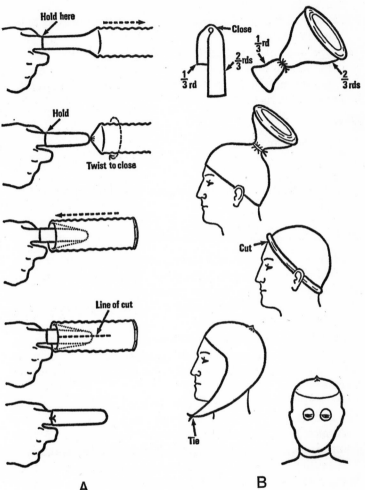

A   B

FIG. 57. THE APPLICATION OF TUBEGAUZ

Shaving equipment
Powder for the limb
Stockinette
Sheet wadding or thick padding of wool if there is likely to be
much swelling
Large bowl of tepid water for soaking the bandages (unless
the bowl is of plastic it should be thinly coated inside with
petroleum jelly to prevent the plaster from sticking to it.)
Plaster of Paris bandages

Tray with:

Tape measure
Blue pencil
Scissors
Plaster shears, knives and scissors if an old plaster needs
removing

Points to be remembered in the application of plaster

Shave the limb, powder it and cover with stockinette or wool.

Hold the limb steady throughout the application and be
careful not to press on the wet plaster.

Trim and turn up the bandages over the edges, polish and
leave smooth.

After the plaster is dry, watch for any blueness of the extremi-
ties and report any complaint of coldness, numbness or pain.
These symptoms would be an indication of interference with the
circulation.

It should be remembered that pressure deadens sensation
and that the skin may be pressed upon and killed.

A nurse must never cut or interfere with plaster. If a patient
complains of the above symptoms a doctor must be informed.

No patient should be sent home with a new plaster on without
being told when to report for examination, and he must be
told to return at once if he is worried or unduly uncomfortable,
if his toes or fingers swell or look blue, feel cold or hurt. A
printed form of instructions should be given to the patient or his
nearest relative before he leaves the hospital.

Index

Index

Glucose, 212, 242
Gluteus maximus, 214
Goitre, 257
Gonorrhoea, 161
Graded milk, 33
Graves' disease, 257
Grey matter, 271
Gynaecology, 262

Haematemesis, 243
Haemoglobin, 222
Haemoptysis, 158
Haemorrhage,
  external, 283
  internal, 86
Haemorrhoids, 225
Hair, 250
  care of, 74
Hamstrings, 214
Hands, 203
  care of, 36
Hanging, 294
Head lice, 27
Healing, process of, 131
Health,
  at school, 10
  of community, 17–25
  of nurses, 35–41
  rules of, 17
  visitor, 7
Health Service, 5
Heart, 217
  disorders of, 219
  failure, 220
Heat, regulation of body, 250
Heating, 21
Heatstroke, 294
Hemiplegia, 276
Heparin, 220
Hernia, 244
Hipjoint, 209
Hodgkin's disease, 226
Home help, 14
Hormones, 253
Hospital management committee, 5
Hospital refuse, 23
Hot water bottles, burns from, 64
House refuse, 23

Human behaviour in illness, 42–4
Human development, 9
Humerus, 203
  fracture of, 288
Hyaline cartilage, 196
Hydrochloric acid, 241
Hygiene,
  of patients, 69–79
  personal, 35–7
Hyperpyrexia, 83
Hyperthyroidism, 257
Hypodermic injection, 99

Ilium, 203
Illness, signs of, 81
Immunity, 140
Immunization, 7
Impetigo, 251
Incontinence, 114
Incontinent patients, 76
Infant, normal, 176
Infant welfare clinic, 7
Infection, 130
  how spread, 138
  prevention of, 139
Infectious diseases,
  caused by impure water, 22
  immunization against, 7
Inferior vena cava, 219
Inflammation, 131
Inhalations, 102
Injections,
  hypodermic, 99
  intramuscular, 101
  intravenous, 129
Inner ear, 267
Innominate bone, 203
Insects, 27
Instruments, care of, 137
Insulin,
  secretion of, 255
  use in diabetes, 256
Intake and output charts, 114
Intervertebral discs, 202
Intestinal obstruction, 244
Intestines, 238
Intramuscular injections, 101
Intravenous injections, 129
Intussusception, 244

THE GENERAL NURSING COUNCIL
FOR ENGLAND AND WALES

LONDON,
W1A 1BA

23 PORTLAND PLACE

TELEPHONES: 01-580 8334
TELEGRAMS: GENURCOUN, LONDON, W.1.

NOTIFICATION OF ADMISSION TO THE INDEX OF   STUDENT NURSES

INDEX NUMBER   0491739   SURNAME   YBESATE

FORENAMES   ROSALINA

TONE VALE HOSPITAL SCHOOL OF NURSING

THIS NOTIFICATION MUST BE RETAINED AND THE
INDEX NUMBER QUOTED ON ALL COMMUNICATIONS
WITH THE GENERAL NURSING COUNCIL.

EXAMINATIONS OFFICER

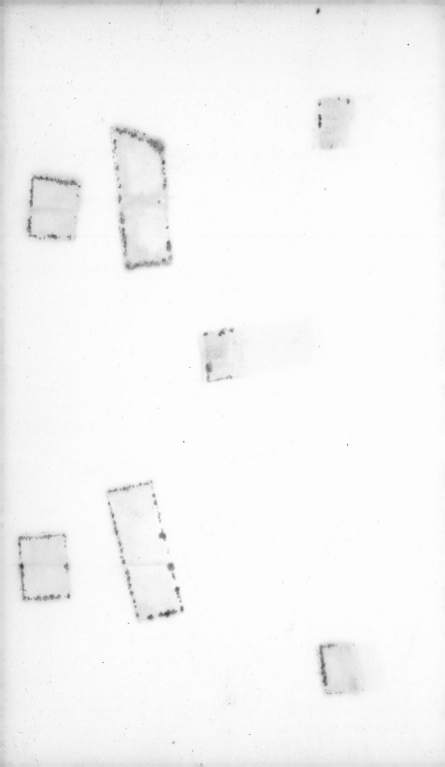